D0008975

THE THIN BOOK BY A FORMERLY FAT PSYCHIATRIST

Books by

THEODORE ISAAC RUBIN, M.D.

Jordi
Lisa and David
In the Life
Sweet Daddy
Platzo and the Mexican Pony Rider
The Thin Book by a Formerly Fat Psychiatrist

THE THIN BOOK BY A FORMERLY FAT PSYCHIATRIST

Theodore Isaac Rubin, M.D.

TRIDENT PRESS New York 1966

Fifth Printing

Library of Congress Catalog Card Number: 66-16181

Published simultaneously in the United States and Canada by Trident Press.

PRINTED IN THE UNITED STATES OF AMERICA

For My Mother and Father

Contents

WHY THIS BOOK 9
FATNESS IS A SICKNESS 11
HOPELESSNESS 14
SOME PEOPLE ARE LUCKY 16
ANY DIET? 19
REALISTIC GOALS 21
PREPARATION FOR FAILURE 23
AMMUNITION FOODS 25
THE PSYCHOLOGY OF TIME 27
SLEEPING BENEFITS 29
VACATIONS AND BINGES 31
MAKING FRIENDS WITH FOOD 34
PSYCHOTHERAPY AND DIETING 36
THE SCALE 39
THE EXERCISE QUESTION—AND THE ANSWER 42
ROUTINES AND SCHEDULES 49
REBELLION, DISCIPLINE, AND FREEDOM 51
A GOOD TIME TO START 53
LET LOVE MOTIVATE YOU 57
SEX, SMOKING, AND SCRUPLES 59
BY THE GROUP 63

THE TEMPTATION OF MENUS 65
VITAMINIZING 67
THE DIETETIC PALATE 68
TAKE TEA FOR COMFORT 70
THE DIET I LIKE BEST 72
MAGIC, MIRACLES, AND MYTHS 76
HELP! I'M STARVED! 78
THE DIET DOLDRUMS 80
HOW TO EAT—GRACIOUSLY 83
ON WALKING AWAY FROM THE TABLE 87
YOUR EVENING EVALUATION 89
APPLES, ASPIRIN, AMOUR 91
THE NIGHT EATERS 94
BEWARE OF FRIENDLY ENEMIES 97
ALLIES TO THE CAUSE 101
YOUR BODY IMAGE 103
SUCCESS—AND MAINTENANCE 106
GLOSSARY 111
QUESTIONS AND ANSWERS 114
LISTS OF AMMUNITION AND COMFORTING FOODS 125
LIST OF "POISON" FOODS 127

Why This Book

I would like to state right from the start that this is not a diet book. This is not a book on the psychodynamics of obesity, and it is certainly not a magic method for losing weight.

As the title says, I have been fat. I have also treated fat people. I have helped myself and I've helped them. I'd like to help you. I believe I can. I feel that fundamentally the problem is one of attitude rather than diet. I also believe that our cause is an entirely worthwhile one. We want to prolong life and to make life worthwhile while we live it. Fatness leads to a shorter life and to one of infirmity—physically, mentally, socially, and even economically. Some of the things you will read here will be totally familiar. Perhaps you've heard them. Perhaps you've even said them. This is no reason to discount them. Perhaps their new and continued emphasis as well as their context here will make them valuable as well as familiar.

The last section of the book consists of questions and answers that have come up, related to the material in the book as well as to miscellaneous matters not discussed in the book. Please save it until you have completed the rest of the book.

The next to the last chapter consists of a short glossary. Please take a few minutes to read it now.

Fatness Is a Sickness

Being fat is a sickness. For our purposes you are fat and sick if you are at all overweight. This applies whether you are mildly sick, i.e., 3 or 4 pounds overweight, or deathly sick, i.e., some 75 or more pounds overweight. Like many sicknesses, neglect will result in the acute becoming chronic and the benign becoming malignant. So, regardless of how overweight and sick you are, please pay heed. Now, you may even call it a psychosomatic sickness. Fat people are anxiety ridden and handle their anxiety through overeating. The latter is a vast oversimplification of the psychiatric part of the condition. The somatic or body part is justified by the presence of the physical lesion or affliction. The lesion here is fat. We're going to call it the "fat tumor" even though it may be spread all over the place. It's just lots of fat, extra fat that strains the heart, blocks the arteries, raises the blood pressure, puts extra weight on veins and joints complicating varicose veins, hemorrhoids, and arthritis just to mention a few. Most of all though it makes you look old and clumsy and ugly and worse yet, indistinguishable from your fellow fat man. All fat people look alike because fat, like leprosy, has a way of ironing out features—just flattening them out and obliterating them. This sickness, like some of its other malignant brothers, shortens life. The physical part of the sickness takes care of that. But it's more than that. This sickness, perhaps like no other, is terribly destructive to one's psychic and social life. Nobody loves a fat man, especially not himself. Now everybody needs love, especially a fatty. If he didn't need love so much, he probably wouldn't be fat in the first place. But enough of that. I promised you—no psychodynamics. Suffice it to say, the fat man has a miserable image of himself, and this affects him enormously—socially, sexually, and economically. Though he may not admit it, he functions largely as a cripple. Worse yet, this kind of cripple evokes contempt rather than sympathy; this situation results in great sensitivity and further crippling of self-esteem and the ability to relate to people. OK, I hope I've motivated you a little bit. I hope I've piqued your vanity. You need motivation. You need it badly. You are destructive, and appealing to your vanity will probably have more effect than appealing to your concern for your health.

All right, you are sick. If you feel sorry for yourself, this is good. You have every reason to feel sorry for yourself. You are a sick person. Why shouldn't you feel sorry for yourself? But don't let's beat up on you. Hating a sick man is no way to treat him. It makes him worse. Self-hate is worst of all since you have to carry it around with you wherever you go, and you already have enough of a load. If you really feel sorry for yourself, you will be gentle to yourself—gentle and caring. But before we get to that, step No. 1 is to admit that you are sick. This is crucial. Only by admitting that you are sick and then accepting this fact without hate will you be in a position to begin to do something about you.

Ask yourself how long you've been fat, how fat, through how many diets and promises? Ask yourself what it's done to you, how it has affected your life and your relationships with other people? If you're ready to admit that overeating and being fat is an obsession, a compulsion, that you are addicted to eating too much food—you are on your way. But none of this kidding. None of this "Oh, I could lose a few pounds," or "All I have to do is make up my mind." Either you are or you aren't a fatty. If you are, it is imperative that you know it, that you make the diagnosis, and that you accept yourself as you are. Now that sounds funny. Accept yourself as you are when you are something you don't want to be. But, and this is a big one, you have been cushioning yourself with fat for years. You have been cushioning yourself against you and the world. Only by accepting you, who and whatever you are, without wasting energy in self-hate, will you be able to change and to grow in a healthier direction.

The biggest enemy of the fat man is self-hate. Self-hate results in pain requiring sedation in the form of food. Real self-concern and real self-pity lead to self-acceptance and the possibility of change. Think about this carefully. Work it over in your mind. When you've made the diagnosis and accept it, you are ready to go on.

Hopelessness

Now that you know you are sick, do you want to get well? Of course you do. But can you? If you are a chronic case, you probably think you can't. Oh, you may tell yourself you can—it's just a question of starting, of making up your mind, and so forth. But deep down where it counts you have the conviction you can't. What we are dealing with here is hopelessness. Deep down, chronically fat people really feel hopeless about the possibility of change. Now this hopelessness is the second biggest enemy of the fat person. Hopelessness is the second best way to maintain the status quo. "I mean why try—it won't work anyway—I may as well eat. What the hell, I'm fifty pounds overweight. Another couple of pounds before I go on a diet isn't going to matter anyway." It isn't going to matter because deep down you feel that no lasting change will ever take place anyway. The rationalizations are endless. Hopelessness and self-hate can be very subtle. You use them again and again as justifications for overeating. Therefore you must be exceedingly wary of them. Remember, hopelessness and self-hate are traps used to maintain your neurotic fat status. The fact is that your illness can be cured. You can get better. Other people have made it—and so can you. But you must be utterly realistic about the struggle. And that is just what it's going to be, a struggle—a long hard struggle for which you must be thoroughly prepared. This preparation and a realistic outlook will give you most needed strength to lick this most malignant killer.

Some People Are Lucky

Again and again we hear this: how lucky some people are. They can eat tremendous amounts of any kind of food at all times of the day and night and not gain weight. The story usually has it that some people are blessed with a very rapid metabolism and immediately burn up everything they eat before it turns to fat. Then, of course, there are fatties. We poor shnooks are cursed with an ultraslow metabolic process and are really fat-manufacturing plants who quite by accident also happen to look human.

Well, it simply ain't so. It is true that people can suffer from hyper- (too much) or hypo- (too little) thyroid function, which can result in a speedy or slow metabolic rate. But let me tell you that most people in this world, and I do mean most, are perfectly normal in this department. A small percentage of the population has a small thyroid dysfunction, but this is almost never enough to account for being a skinny or a fatty. There are serious and severe diseases of thyroid and other endocrine (i.e., hormone glands such as the pituitary) functions. But these are rare; where they do occur, there are almost always concomitantly present plenty of symptoms besides too much or too little weight. More often than not, the physician will readily note these symptoms and will initiate the tests necessary to ascertain their origin. If your doctor has not put you through the various tests for thyroid function (basal metabolism rate, blood iodine, blood cholesterol, and so forth), it is because he sees no symptoms that would indicate endocrine dysfunction; he believes that you are a simple fatty. If you are convinced that you are suffering from fatness and nothing else—(believe me, that's enough)—we are ready to go on. But if you are not convinced and prefer to externalize your problem to a source other than your own immediate responsibility (like to your maverick glands), then please take action at once. Have a discussion with your doctor, and by all means have a thorough endocrine checkup. This may cost several hundred dollars but if you come away convinced it will be well worth it. As we said earlier, it is imperative to our continuing success that you realize that you are sick and that you—not your glands—take responsibility for your sickness and your cure. The sickness we speak of here is fatness—simple fatness. Its origin is simple, too. For your size and physical output of energy, you have been taking in too many calories via the various substances called "food." The cure is equally simple. You must eat less food or food that contains fewer calories. In any case you must ingest fewer calories and must eventually balance your calorie input and your energy output. You cannot do this successfully, let alone sustain it over a lifetime, if you persist in envying mythical glandular wonder children. Your trouble is your appetite, not your glands. Therefore, take whatever steps that are necessary to ascertain this and to convince yourself once and for all so that we can be on our realistic way.

Any Diet?

The diet doesn't matter. Perhaps this sounds funny, but there are any number of good diets and practically all of them work. See your doctor and ask him what is safe for you. See a doctor in whom you have faith. But much more important, see a man who has faith in you and in your ability to help yourself—without pills.

Please, no pills, no "medical aids" unless, and *only* if, your doctor prescribes them (and then strictly in accordance with his directions)—this is very important! The results must come from you and you must know that they came from you, not from some magic medicine. You need self-esteem desperately and pills will destroy it. From the very start you must convince yourself of a basic truth: if you are to be successful, that success must come from you. You, not pills, must be responsible, and you must feel that responsibility and the subsequent feel of self-accomplishment. If you are robbed of that feeling, any initial success will only result in capitulation later on. Remember—we are engaged in a most difficult campaign, fighting a most pervasive enemy. If victory is to be ours, we must use every means at our command.

Do ask your doctor if a crash diet of a week's duration is compatible with your state of health. The loss of a few pounds can be a good morale booster as a start.

Realistic Goals

Fat people tend to be expansive and grandiose. Perhaps this is a reaction to their basic insecurity. In any case, they tend to operate in an "all or nothing" way. If you operate this way, you are very likely to set exorbitant goals. This can be very dangerous—for discouragement, especially early in the game, can be completely devastating.

Now we are not suggesting that you minimize the problem. Being 70 pounds overweight is being 70 pounds overweight and there's no point kidding about it. Neither the scale nor your doctor is going to lie to you. We don't suggest that you do. A 70-pound "fat tumor" is 70 pounds no matter how it is distributed and no matter how you kid yourself. But thinking in terms of 70 pounds from the beginning is also unrealistic. We must think and work in terms of practical working units. Also, different stages of the game may require slight modifications.

Goal 1 is to indicate to yourself that it can be done. That is why we recommend an immediate crash diet designed to help you get rid of 10 percent of the total weight you want to lose. Goal 1 in a 70-pound "fat tumor" would be a loss of 7 pounds. This initial loss will be an important morale booster. Now we do not recommend starvation. Your doctor can advise you about one or another crash diets. Do not starve! There are crash diets in which you can eat. It is likely that your doctor will recommend a high-protein, very low-carbohydrate diet. That is fine. Remember to drink lots of water. Constipation is often an initial response to serious dieting and can be both painful and demoralizing.

After this initial goal has been achieved, you may feel "OK, so what is 7 out of 70—practically nothing." But 7 out of 70 is 10 percent—not even banks pay that. This is a wonderful accomplishment and you are on your way. We must operate in terms of working units while keeping the large goal in mind. At the beginning, 10 percent of the "tumor" is not a bad working goal; and it should give you a great sense of accomplishment, and even pleasure, to visualize that gross "tumor" spread over the entire body shrinking and receding and eventually disappearing completely. Later on, 20 percent of the "tumor" is a good goal. No single goal unit should exceed 20 percent. This is enough to conceptualize satisfactorily. For example, let's say your "tumor" is down to 30 pounds. Six pounds is then the next good goal to contemplate.

Preparation for Failure

It is exceedingly important for you to know from the beginning that you will have failures. This knowledge is essential to keep you in complete contact with reality. Reality is absolutely necessary if you are to avoid disappointment and future self-destructiveness. Disappointment will inevitably fan up self-hate and hopelessness, which will then lead a downhill course to resignation and helplessness. This is especially true if you are a perfectionist. If you expect perfect dieting, you are already on your way to a massive failure since your initial failures will lead to massive self-hate. You will have failures. Be sure of this and be prepared for them. If you face this fact squarely, the total venture will be a success.

Now, how do we prepare for failure? Failure is not black or white. Failure comes in different degrees, and a 50 percent failure is not the same as a 100 percent or total failure. But even with total failure, the course can still be passed. Now, how is it possible to fail realistically, practically, and even in the eventual service of success?

Let us say that you are breaking your diet. You are on an eating binge. I do not mean a reward period nor do I mean eating "ammunition" food, both of which we will speak of later. I mean a simple destructive binge like a high carbohydrate jag—for example, a couple of peanut butter sandwiches and a double chocolate malted. Now to any extent—and I mean to any extent whatever—that you can limit this binge, to that extent you are mitigating failure, fighting despair later, and helping to recoup precious ground immediately after the retreat. Even in failure, keep success in mind. Try, try, try to limit the scope of the failure. Three-quarters of a malted is better than a full one, and half is better yet. Leave over half of that peanut butter sandwich. It's hard—hard as hell. You've had the taste, and all your past conditioning implores you to go on. But settle for what you have had and stop.

This kind of control will indicate to you that you do have a capacity for self-control, for frustration tolerance, for success, and for life and happiness. All right, the binge is now over. Do not hate or chastise yourself or even feel guilty. Guilt is a cheap commodity, a poor substitute for responsibility. You are not guilty. You are responsible—don't sell that responsibility cheaply. You did it. Now what can you do about it? How come the break? Were you anxious? Depressed? Isn't this an old habit—depression, eating, then more depression? Learn what you can from the failure. A good general adds to his fund of knowledge even in defeat. Now what went well? Was control better? Was it implemented faster? Which or how much food didn't you eat? Self-praise helps.

Ammunition Foods

Now let us talk about ammunition food, that is, food that helps to prevent failure and to limit it. It is too much for you to hope to succeed in eating your three diet meals and nothing else. Such an approach is not realistic or in keeping with a long-standing way of life. If I know you, you are a nosher. But there are ways of noshing. There are cheese, nuts, crackers, pizzas, and so forth, all very tasty and extremely destructive.

Then there are ammunition foods. These are foods that satisfy both appetite and our purpose. These are foods that you can eat in any quantity, foods that you must always keep in the house. I am sure that you will find a favorite few. Let me list some that *I* like: sour pickles (not sweet and sour but dill pickles, that is, kosher pickles, the kind one finds in Jewish delicatessens), celery stalks, cooked mushrooms, sauerkraut, strawberries, tomatoes, brussels sprouts, carrot sticks, lettuce leaves, cucumbers, cauliflower, and so forth.

Then there are "emergency" foods. OK, you're under attack. Things are tough today. Worse—

you're about to have an attack. You must have something sweet and you're beyond your day's dietary allowance. Have some low-calorie chocolate pudding and low-calorie cream whip. The combination totals 65 calories. Or have a portion of low-calorie gelatin dessert and cream whip (totalling 40 calories) or half a cantaloupe or tea and animal cookies (six—no more). Or, if more solid food is necessary, have a meatball patty or a small steak. You should always have ammunition foods and emergency foods on hand. But, remember, if you go wild (I mean banana-split wild), then split the split and leave half of it over—or a third or even leave a drop. If you just can't, then (as in the "rape is inevitable" story) sit back and enjoy it—but do not give up. Begin again at once—not with chastisement but with greater preparation for tough periods. Try to find out what caused the break—fatigue, depression, too many bills, income tax time. In the future, be wary of such times and be especially kind to yourself, but not with "tumor" feeding food. In any case, begin again at once and think well of yourself for beginning again rather than resigning in hopelessness.

One banana split is an awful lot of calories, but it isn't what got you to this state in the first place. Likewise, it will not destroy your newly discovered self-interest in your state of health. You got this way through years of bad eating habits, so settle down again to learning some good ones and don't be thrown by bumps in the road. The road winds on and eventually straightens out, and you can make it if you desire. Since you are reading this book, we assume that you do desire!

The Psychology of Time

Time is on your side. It is important that you make friends with it and use it in your behalf. Chances are that the fatter you are the less able you've been to get along with time. You probably have great difficulty waiting—waiting for anything. Yet if you learn to wait, time will serve you well.

Now it took a long time to become a fat person and to establish yourself in that role. It will take time to become thin. It will take even more time to establish your thinness as a way of life, that is, to remain thin.

Taking your time in getting thin is most important. First, it gives your body an opportunity to acclimate itself to its new dimensions. The stomach has a chance to shrink. The skin has a chance to tighten. Instead of a thin empty bag you will be a thin person. But much more important, your psychology regarding yourself, and yourself in relation to food, will have had a chance at permanent healthy change. By contrast, let us start with the proposition that a miracle pill is on the market. You take the pill, go to sleep, and wake up thin. Are you then a thin person? You look thin. But you are still a fat person in your image of yourself and in your way of handling yourself vis-à-vis food. It is the time and work and struggle involved in getting thin that will reestablish your image and your eating habits as well as your morale and your sense of self-reliance and responsibility for self. This responsibility for self is an extremely important item. Like other neurotic people the fat person has come to feel that he is a will-o'-the-wisp, subject to outside and uncontrollable forces and events—in this case an insatiable and unfulfilled appetite. Taking responsibility for self is crucial in restoring a sense of equilibrium and ownership to oneself. Time is necessary. It is necessary in order to acclimate yourself to this new way of life. It takes time to shrink a stomach, to shrink an appetite, to place food on the periphery of your existence rather than to focus on it as the central kernel of your life. It takes time to substitute other interests and activities for eating, to invest emotions in areas other than eating, and to socialize without the stimulation and necessity of chronic, constant food binges.

I can understand your impatience for results and your anticipation of a less stringent diet. But our goals are extravagant. We want lasting results, not quick ones. We must achieve a reorientation to eating. This takes time.

Sleeping Benefits

Sleep is another very important ally. Being tired is demoralizing. This can be a subtle chronic process or it can be quite acute, just blatant fatigue. With fat people the result of either type is the same. When their morale is low, they eat. But the problem goes deeper than that. When people are well-rested and have ample energy, there is no extraordinary need to seek energy via food. When people are tired they naturally gravitate to food to replenish their supply of energy. Now this process of energy depletion and refueling is always considerably amplified in fat people. Being tired destroys morale, kindles pessimism about oneself, destroys resolve, and leads to the rationalization that food (just this once) will make you feel better. There is the additional fact that adequate sleep will lead to fewer waking hours—less time to eat. Now I do not advocate staying in bed all day or lounging about day in and day out. But ample sleep is an absolute requirement for success. Each individual has a fairly good idea of his particular sleep requirements, and it is extremely important to listen to oneself on this score. Do get enough sleep to feel well-rested.

I would like to point out that people need people, and that this is especially true of fat people. Therefore if your sleep pattern is in keeping with the rest of the people in your household, you are one step ahead of the game. Otherwise it is a good idea, especially at the beginning, to reestablish that pattern. What I'm trying to say is simply this: If you are tired but ignore your fatigue and stay up late watching television alone, you are in an exceedingly vulnerable position. Go to sleep when everybody else does and, if necessary and possible, get additional sleep besides.

Vacations and Binges

I want to talk about units again but not about the practical working units I discussed before. These are much larger units. Let's call them goal units. I feel that goal units can be from 10 to 20 pounds but not more than 20 pounds. This means that a 60-pound "tumor" can, for example, be segmented into six 10-pound units or three 20-pound units. The choice of unit size should depend on what you think is practically possible for you in terms of prolonged disciplined eating. If the strain of this discipline is great, then don't be a hero; decide on a smaller unit.

Now, why segment the "tumor"? Why not do the whole bit in one long burst? Isn't it more difficult to diet, vacation from dieting, and then go back to dieting? Because this is precisely what I am suggesting—that you diet until you arrive at the end of a goal unit, then vacation from dieting for a month, and then return to the diet. Yes, this is hard. But in learning that it can be done, your morale and your sense of self-control will improve and you will be better able to resume dieting at any time in your life if the necessity arises.

There are additional, more important reasons, however; for instance, the matter of incentive (as in practical working-unit goals) and the matter of acclimating to a maintenance diet. First, let me say that a vacation does not mean going hog wild and I use the word *hog* advisedly. A vacation from dieting after a goal unit has been reached means going on a maintenance diet. A maintenance diet is the diet you will ultimately go on for the rest of your life in order to maintain your weight without gain or loss. We will speak more of the maintenance diet in a later chapter. I only wish to say now that it is extremely important to acclimate to this maintenance diet as soon as possible and over as long a period as possible. Success in acclimating to the maintenance diet will ultimately result in your sustaining at the end of your dieting the weight loss you will have achieved. These "vacations" are all important in getting your body and psyche used to the nondieting period—the major period in your life and the most difficult one. It is hard to lose weight, but it is much more difficult to sustain the loss. Losing weight is dramatic; there is change, excitement, stimulation, and attention. Sustaining the weight loss means maintaining the status quo undramatically, without calling attention to oneself. "Vacationing" will be all-important in getting used to this toughest period of all. So choose a goal unit, and "vacation" for one month after you achieve each goal unit.

"Vacationing" also has a very good effect physiologically. The food deprivation is less drastic. The acclimatization of the body is gradual. This means that drastic changes, which are unkind to the body, will not take place. But primarily we avoid producing the empty bag man. I mean the thin man with a fat man's appetite and a fat man's outlook toward food, a man who is only looking forward to his diet's end so that he can start eating gluttonously all over again. So do it slowly—slowly—slowly—with goal units of no more than 20 pounds and with vacations after each goal unit. We will segment the "tumor" and segment it again and again until it is gone and stays gone.

Above all, do not confuse a prolonged and chronic binge with a vacation. The former is impulsive and lacks planning and control. It is not designed to maintain but to gain, and it becomes a destructive enterprise. The latter, namely segmenting and vacationing, is planned, is under your control, maintains your weight without gain, and is entirely constructive. So no rationalizations, please! A binge is a binge and must be handled accordingly. A vacation is the result of serious work and part of the serious process of "tumor" removal.

Making Friends with Food

Yes, dieting is going to help you make friends with food. I know this sounds paradoxical but it's true. You haven't been friends for years—you and food. You hate food because of what it has done to you and you attack it that way. You chop away at it indiscriminately. You have lost the taste for quality and have become primarily interested in quantity, amassing as much food as possible as quickly as possible. Sometimes you pretend to care. You make critical comments but you continue to eat as if your life depends on it and you don't like it at all. Nobody likes the item or person he is dependent on since it is a reminder of his own inadequacy and infirmity. In this respect you are no different from the drug addict and his dependency and hatred for the addicting drug. This is also too often true of the neurotically handicapped person and his wheelchair or crutch. They have a strange relationship —one of dependency and hatred.

But food is not responsible for your condition. It is you and the way you have come to use food. I feel that getting thin will restore your mutual self-respect—you and the stuff you eat. Eating less food and eating less ravenously will give you the chance to observe and to dignify what you are eating. Peculiar as it may sound, the fat man is simply not a gourmet. He is almost always a most indiscriminate eater. Eating great quantities and great varieties of food simply does not permit discreet tasting and the subtle pleasures derived therefrom. I was recently in a fine Chinese restaurant where I had the chance to observe two men eating. One was very fat and the other normally thin. The fat man seemed to eat with gusto. But as I watched carefully, the fat man heaped foods from every platter on his plate and with seeming unawareness mixed them together and ate them. He shoveled this great mélange down as quickly as possible, and I'm sure he could not differentiate one Chinese delicacy from another. Our thin friend ate slowly from one platter at a time, allowing himself to partake of the individual flavor of each dish before proceeding to the next. It was as if the fat man's taste for food had been obliterated in his rush to fill his stomach more and more and still more.

You will reestablish respect for food by getting thin, or establish it if you've never had it before. You know what damage excessive eating can create, having been in that territory yourself. But for the first time, or the first time in a long time, your finer sensibilities will have been restored. Each morsel will become meaningful as you become discriminating and sophisticated in your new-found taste sensitivity. You will have made a friend of food. A compulsive routine will have changed to pleasurable activity free of guilt, thereby adding sweetness to your life.

Psychotherapy and Dieting

Psychotherapy is almost impossibly ineffectual without motivation. It is the rare therapist who can motivate a patient to get psychiatric help and to remain long enough to be helped if the patient does not so desire. But people who are motivated to get help for themselves through psychiatric treatment can be motivated to diet. Through psychotherapy, especially analytic psychotherapy, such people can become sufficiently interested in themselves—constructively—to really want to do something about their fatness. More important, they can work toward a better understanding of what set of psychodynamics made them fat in the first place and what kept them fat. To understand one's symptoms through insight and the comprehension of one's emotions is invaluable. Such understanding offers the possibility of removing whatever it is that caused this pernicious symptom in the first place and the possibility of freedom and growth in many other areas as well.

But it is not my intention to sell you psychiatric treatment. As I have just said, the patient must do that for himself. I do not believe that all fat people need psychiatric treatment in order to get thin. People with self-motivation who want to change can get thin without professional help.

In this particular issue the symptom is often even more serious than the disease that caused it. Not only can the patient die if the symptom—fatness—is not removed at once, but the symptom itself becomes an almost autonomous sickness. What I'm trying to say is this: A poor concept of one's self in relation to one's self and one's fellows may lead to fatness. But fatness invariably leads to even more disturbing and aberrant ways of seeing one's self in relation to the rest of the world. Breaking up this vicious cycle at any point is invaluable. Tackling it at the fatness level may not only be the best and most dramatic approach, it may also be the only approach.

Also, may I stress that in no circumstance can we psychoanalyze a dead patient. If the patient is motivated, we must first save his life; then, if he is so inclined, he will have the opportunity to seek psychiatric treatment. If the patient is not motivated, if he cannot get started, or if he is suffering from malignant fatness (such as a "tumor" of more than 100 pounds and symptoms like compulsive all-night eating), then he needs psychiatric treatment and may even require immediate hospitalization.

Night eating, that is, compulsive eating several times during the night, is often an indication of what I call malignant fatness. Even the sternest or most supportive medical treatment in or out of a hospital setting will not produce sustained changes in these cases unless psychotherapy by a highly skilled practitioner is also instituted.

Then there are people, fortunately not too many, in whom too drastic or too rapid removal of the symptom (with almost complete deprivation of food) will result in the onset of severe anxiety and depression, often masked by a quick and complete loss of appetite. This is a very serious condition and must be treated immediately by a trained psychiatrist. Here again, may I stress the value of a medical consultation before you get started. If your physician has doubts, a psychiatric consultation may be in order. If after getting started, you feel overanxious, jumpy, nervous, moody, or blue, or if you experience mood swings, then it may be that your diet is too drastic and that you need help. Don't be a hero. If you need professional help, get it. It may be the best thing you've ever done for yourself, not only in losing weight but in opening doors to wonderful possibilities in your life of which you have never even dreamed.

More often than not, the fat man has covered many of his assets with layers of fat; he needs help in putting himself in touch with the happiness that he no longer knows exists.

The Scale

Let's talk about the instrument that brings us good news.

Compulsive use of the scale early in the game (and I've known people who've jumped on and off some twenty times a day) can be quite discouraging. The patient is terribly eager for change and awfully disappointed and discouraged when there is no such indication on his scale after every few hours of dieting. But I know that you will use the scale; it would be inhuman to expect you to do otherwise. However, regardless of the diet you go on, don't expect big changes immediately. They just won't occur, not even with complete starvation. There will be early changes, especially with a crash diet, but these will not occur quickly enough to satisfy most people's impatience. Also, an initial weight loss of any significance will probably be due to an early loss of water. The intake of less food means less salt in the body to bind the water. This process varies from person to person but can make for some disquieting fluctuations. So in the very beginning, the scale may indicate nothing at all. Later on, with early water shifts, your weight may go up and down quite a lot until things level off. Don't blame your scale or yourself; things will level off and progress will be made. In the not too distant future, your scale will show steady changes in the downward direction.

Of course your choice of scale is important; after all it is the only instrument you will use in this vital medical endeavor. I believe that the best scale is the type you find in a doctor's office. It need not be a professional model, but it ought to be patterned after the doctor's scale you've seen time and again. This is the scale in which balances, coarse and fine, must be adjusted to get one's weight. It may be a little more expensive than the usual bathroom variety, but since you will use it all your life it will be well worth its price. Several companies manufacture them, and it pays to get as solid a model as possible. Make sure that your scale stands on a level floor when you set it up. Also, it is important for accuracy that you weigh yourself at the same time of day and at the same time in relation to your meals and bowel movements. And of course you must weigh yourself in the same clothed or unclothed condition. If you are undressed, try (again almost impossible) not to look in the mirror every day, because you will not see any significant change for weeks. You can do without an extra discouragement at this point.

After several months of dieting the scale will be useful to determine the efficacy of your diet; at this point you should check back with your doctor if necessary. I'm not talking about plateaus or periods of doldrums. I'll speak more about these later.

The most important use of the scale will be during the maintenance period. From the time you reach the ultimate goal and for the rest of your life, it will be necessary to weigh yourself every day. I'll tell you more about this in the chapter on maintenance. Suffice it to say here that these daily weight measurements will be one of the few concessions you will make to your former fat-man status. But since you will use the scale forever, be sure to get a good sturdy instrument on which the values can be read at eye level—even though the pot belly that blocks your downward view is on its way to oblivion.

The Exercise Question—and the Answer

There are people who will have you believe that you can trim off the fat "tumor" with exercise. The variety of exercises recommended is infinite. Massage treatments of all kinds are also advocated. Exercise alone simply will not do it! Massages, while they may be pleasant, will have even less effect. You may achieve some small redistribution of the fat "tumor" through the exclusive use of exercise, but chances are excellent that you will retain your weight within 5 pounds. Some people may even gain weight through an increase in appetite and food intake and a change in water balance. Yet people will often embark on the most strenuous course of exercise rather than go on a diet. Why? There are two main reasons. First, the obvious: Fatties like to eat, need to eat, and will do anything to avoid giving up a morsel of food. The appeal of exercise fads is obvious. Fatties can go on eating and at the same time can continue to delude themselves that they are doing something valuable for themselves. But the second reason is more important and worth understanding because it affects your total effort (diet plus exercise). One of the most difficult things about losing weight is that you are required *not* to do something—in this case the *not* refers to eating. We are not a nation of waiters, and I'm afraid that patience is not one of our more common virtues. Generally, we are oriented to accomplish things by doing rather than by not doing, and we do not take kindly to what feels like passivity in the service of attaining a goal. Now exercise has the appeal of "doing," while not eating bears the stigma of "not doing." Let me tell you something, however. Refraining from eating —not eating—is an extremely active process. Dieting involves self-control and self-management and is an investment in self-accomplishment and the building of responsibility for self. Dieting represents all this and more and as such is a very active process indeed. Yes, passivity can be a most active, energetic and worthwhile process. I think that Mahatma Gandhi demonstrated this point admirably. While I do not recommend Gandhi-like fasts, I do want to stress the fact that you are used to *doing* and in this situation you will be *not doing;* but I daresay that not doing can take more energy, more courage, and more dedication.

Do exercises have any role in our work? Of course they do. But the role of exercise is minor compared with that of dieting. Exercise has its importance—but the central core of our effort is dieting. Exercise remains an adjunct while you stay away from "poison" foods.

Now what about this valuable adjunct?

First and of extreme importance is the warning

that no exercise, and I mean not even the mildest, should be undertaken without a thorough-going physical examination and clearance by your doctor. This is especially true for fat people who have been grossly overweight for extended periods of time. Among this group, examination sometimes reveals high blood pressure as well as cardiac conditions. Should you be cleared for mild exercise, please remember to keep it mild and never to let it outstrip your weight. You will of course be able to do a little more as your weight approaches normal.

Your doctor and specialists in physical education, physical therapy, and physical rehabilitation, as well as many excellent books, will be able to give you suggestions regarding mild exercises. There are some fine books on isometric exercises, which employ the method of prolonged contraction of muscles for short intervals of time; for example, keeping one's belly sucked in for half a minute several times a day. Isometrics seem easy but can be quite effective if properly used. These books will be best used, however, only after you are well within sight of your normal weight. My two favorite exercises are walking and swimming, and I am not against golf, table tennis, and bowling after you have lost much of the "tumor." Be apprised, however, that even walking can be very strenuous for the fat man, especially in hot weather. So don't go overboard. Limit yourself to a few blocks at first and then gradually increase to a few miles as you acclimate to movement.

Now what about the value of exercise? Some experts in physiology say that it is completely without value and that it can even be detrimental to our ultimate goal. They say that the calories expended in exercise are of minor importance and that the resultant increase in appetite usually results in an increase in calorie intake far beyond that expended. In short, they say that exercise will not make you thin and may even make you fat.

Other experts make claims for another factor, however. They say that exercise has a physiological effect beyond and much more important than that of weight redistribution or intake and output of caloric energy. They claim that moderate but regular exercise tends to keep the metabolism moving along regularly so that calories are used up far beyond the amount required by the exercise itself. They say that this is particularly evident in sedentary people who do not use caloric energy and have also developed a sluggish metabolism. In these people exercise serves as a catalyst. As a utilizer of calories its function is minor, but its effect on the metabolic rate, the rate at which calories are burned up, is major. In short, exercise keeps the motor tuned up, running smoothly, and running steadily at a good clip. Perhaps my opinion is colored by wishful thinking. While I am a physician and know something of physiology, I am certainly not an expert. But I will say this—there seems to be much in human metabolism that we still do not understand and in my experience sensible controlled exercise in conjunction with dieting does help. I have experimented both with myself and with patients; and the rate of weight loss is increased about 10 percent with exercise. How much of this result is physiological and how much of it is psychological I do not know. I have never subscribed to the psychological/physiological dichotomy anyway. It is all happening in one body, and without one there is no other. But what about some of the stuff we have come to call psychological effects?

I think that here is where we begin to see some very important aspects of exercise. By exercising you have the opportunity to *do* rather than to do by *not doing*. Therefore, exercise and enjoy it in the knowledge that you are participating in a constructive enterprise involving your own personal progress. You can thus have the dual satisfaction of passive activity and active activity offered by the combination of dieting and exercising.

There is another very important aspect of exercise for the fat man or woman. The fat woman has, to a great extent, lost touch with her physical self. She has come to think of herself as a physical nonentity. She looks upon herself as a glob, a mattress, a receptacle for food, an object of ridicule and derision and above all self-hate. Her body has come to represent and to be symbolic of her social and other interpersonal failures. It has come to be her symbol of social resignation. As such, in her emotional view of herself she has put as much distance as possible between herself and her body. This sounds funny—I mean, how can you separate yourself from your body? Physically you can't. Psychologically you can and do. How? By no longer having a good feeling for your body, by no longer enjoying the feelings that come from your physical self, by attributing to old age the feelings which are in fact the result of old fat.

Please do not confuse the pleasure of eating with bodily pleasure. Your eating is not a pleasure. It has become a compulsion and the only way you can feel some small measure of false comfort and security. Exercise helps one to feel one's body. In using one's body (and it's amazing how much disuse a fat man's body can endure), one begins to feel it again and to enjoy the feeling of it again. This is especially true when changes—healthy, flattering changes—are taking place. As you get thin you will feel better about your body and your image of it will slowly change. Exercise will enhance this change in feeling and will accelerate the process. As you exercise you will have an increasing awareness of the "feel" of you as a physical human being and of the healthy, attractive changes taking place. You will come to realize that many of the aches and creaks and physical limitations you have felt have not been old age at all. While it is true that you are not getting younger, you are getting thinner and getting to be you.

Exercise also tends to be relaxing. Mild exercise is an excellent tranquilizer. Using up energy in this way helps to quell anxiety stemming from the deprivation of that old neurotic defense—food. But exercising to relax and getting mildly tired does not mean exhaustion. Do not get exhausted. Great fatigue will lead to eating. If you are tired—sleep! And evaluate. You may be overdoing it. In exercising, age, weight, physical condition, and recent exercise history are all important factors in determining just how much you can do. Establishing an exercise routine (fifteen minutes a day) is very valuable, but it should be a routine commensurate with your needs and limitations. Initially, exercise may be difficult. Once the routine is established, however, it can be quite enjoyable. You can get thin without exercising, but if you do, you will be missing a most valuable morale booster and adjunct to your diet.

Routines and Schedules

We have just spoken of routine exercising. At the same time, of course, you will also have been establishing routine eating. Later on I shall tell you more about the value of routine in eating every meal—that is, in making sure that you do not skip meals. But what about the establishment of routine? Isn't this rather compulsive, lacking in spontaneity? Perhaps. Routinizing eating and exercising, putting oneself on a therapeutic regimen, has a somewhat compulsive quality. But remember that if this is compulsion it is being used in the service of health. It is being used to combat the overeating compulsion, a true compulsion based on an almost pure function of anxiety. Our routine is not a result of anxiety and sickness but rather a quest for health.

Routine is important, and I do not mean only routine eating and routine exercising and routine sleeping and resting. In general it will help make it easier and help you to succeed ultimately if you are at loose ends as little as possible during the therapeutic course. If you are engaged in work that absorbs you a good deal of the time, fine. If you have hobbies, fine. In fact, try not to have excess free time on your hands. Plan the use of your time as much as you possibly can. Weekends are particularly dangerous. Plan them carefully. If you do not have social commitments, be especially careful to fill in the time. Do your "do-it-yourself" chores, your fixing, painting, sewing, cleaning, bathing, reading, telephone calling, and so forth, but don't mope around. If the ways in which you use your time over the week become routinized, so much the better. A sensible non-fatiguing schedule that leaves little free time for ruminating and temptation is most important.

Therefore, I strongly suggest that you make a time study of what your weeks have been like before you begin this serious project. Analyze your activities and the amount of time they take. Then sit down and plan yourself a practical working schedule. By "working" I mean one that works, one that is not impossible to fulfill. This schedule can be a valuable asset in the campaign you are about to launch. Remember to leave yourself adequate time to eat. Eating regularly is important. But more about that later on. Plan your schedule, plan it carefully, and plan one you can keep.

Rebellion, Discipline, and Freedom

While some of us do rather well with routine, especially routines of the constructive variety, most of us are sensitive to coercion to some extent. Unfortunately, indiscriminate eating—eating wildly—is sometimes confused with freedom, especially freedom from coercion. In the same state of confusion, sticking to a diet and a constructive regimen is felt as coercive, dictatorial, and constrictive. Often all this is completely unconscious and only makes itself felt by inhibiting the dieting and causing irritation, rebellion, and often resignation. "I just can't do it and that's that, so I'll live a few years less" is only too common a statement.

Well, make no mistake about it. Wild eating is not a function of freedom. It is a result of compulsion—unyielding, blind, indiscriminate compulsion. It could not be more lacking in freedom. It is the antithesis of freedom. Please remember this fact and digest it. On the other hand, the decision to diet, to establish a constructive routine, is born of the freedom to make an important, self-constructive, responsible adult decision for oneself. It takes freedom to make the free choice of doing something for oneself. Of course, you will not get over your sensitivity to discipline, even self-discipline, immediately. It would take several years of analysis to fully cope with this kind of problem. But—you can be aware of the difficulty and you can be wary of destructive rationalizations, hopelessness, and resignation.

Of course there is a realistic curtailment in what you can and cannot do. But this is an adult curtailment based on an adult decision—an adult sense of responsibility with adult attainments and life-saving goals in the offing. With an understanding of your sensitivity to coercion, the real deprivations and limitations entailed by your diet will have a constructive effect.

A Good Time to Start

The Talmud says—If I am not for myself, who will be? If I am only for myself, who am I? If not now, when? Dieting is for yourself and for your loved ones since they would like you to be around for a while; if you are fat, the time to do something about it is now. But now is not necessarily this second. Our "now" ought to be a real one—a point of departure that will really be the start of something good.

Like the invasion of Europe, D Day ought to be chosen with care. First there is no point in starting at all if you haven't made the diagnosis—that is, if you haven't come to the realization that you are sick. But that is not enough. You must have come to the point where you accept your sickness and yourself with your sickness. You are suffering from fatness. You do not hate yourself. On the contrary, you are kindly disposed to yourself and you are about to do something very nice for you.

But first, are you thoroughly prepared? How is your motivation? Are you convinced that fatness has in fact made you vulnerable to the complications of small ailments of all kinds and highly susceptible to the onslaught of chronic debilitating diseases? Are you convinced that only relative youth and luck have fended off paralyzing strokes, crippling heart attacks, and arteriosclerosis? Are you aware that because of your fatness routine surgery would become serious and major and that major surgery might not be possible at all—even if it were a life-saving necessity? Are you aware that fat has served the purpose of an ugly mask, that it has destroyed your individuality and made you a cipher—just another member of the fat population? Are you aware that fatness has destroyed your sex appeal and made you look older, somewhat like a buffoon whom people are initially inclined not to take seriously in any area or on any level? Are you aware that you have to "prove yourself" ten times more than a thin man socially and in business and that this has worn you out both physically and psychologically? In short, are you truly tired of sustaining the role of the family freak or the crowd's fat man? If so, then you are adequately motivated to change the status quo, to begin to come out of your fatness, and to grow as a healthy human being.

But pick a good time to start. Important enterprises, and this is a most important one, deserve the very best kind of send-off. Here, the best time means that which will give you every advantage in overcoming initial inertia and temptation. Start on a morning when you are particularly well-rested and feeling good and know that you will be fairly busy. Have your house cleared of excess poison food for several days previously. Orient your family or the people you live with, and have plenty of ammunition food, comforting food, and emergency supplies on hand and easy to reach. Ideally, the next several days should be days of pleasant but well-organized routine—not weekends of unplanned "free" time with nothing to do but eat. Your routine ought to include getting out of the house, but not to eating places. Ordinary work days are fine—usually much better than vacation days—but guard carefully against excess work and excess fatigue. These should be busy days but "take-it-easy" days. During these early days frequent naps are valuable indeed since you will probably initially get attacks of fatigue, which increase temptation a great deal. If weather is important to you, pick a cheerful sunny day to start, but please don't use this or other excuses to procrastinate indefinitely. Remember it's your life that's in the balance. Fat people, like all neurotics, have developed a feeling of omnipotence as a reaction to their inadequacy. It's always the next guy who has the heart attack and dies. Well, there's a good chance that he's fat, too, and the next guy can be you, so wise up and get started. I hope that you have picked a time as free as possible of excessive pressures, business and otherwise. Do avoid such pressures as much as possible, especially at the beginning.

Remember that you are a sick person undertaking a most difficult operation—obliteration of a dangerous "tumor." This enterprise requires every break you can give it, and only you can give it the breaks it needs. Do not undertake other large self-interest tasks at this time. This is not the time to give up smoking. That will come at another time. This is not the time to incur added pressure. You are about to be engaged in an activity which is difficult enough. Don't be grandiose! Don't undertake more than one difficult job at a time. I know and you know that smoking, eating, and talking are related, but this is all the more reason not to attempt to completely curtail oral activity at this time. I am not advocating that you take up smoking. If you haven't been a smoker, chances are you are a talker. Talk all you want. But if you are addicted to tobacco and want to give it up, do it after your dieting days are over.

Fat, grandiose people have a tendency to undertake too much at the same time in an all or nothing approach. It goes like this, "OK, I'm really going to improve in all things—no food, no smoking, exercises, new sex habits—I'm changing me over, now, completely." Don't do it. You will fail and you may become severely depressed. Dieting is enough for now—plenty, believe me.

Well, if all is in order, and I assume that you have seen your doctor and chosen your diet, then you are ready to begin. Remember, pick a day carefully. It's your day and from that day there will be many good ones in which you will be working in your behalf as well as for those people in your life who really love and need you.

Let Love Motivate You

Motivation is one of the most difficult items to generate. For people who need psychiatric help there is a truism that coming in to treatment is half the battle. This is one truism I believe in. Why? Because coming to the doctor's office is evidence of that all-important item—motivation. Motivating patients to do something about themselves in order to get well is one thing that still defies us. Motivation must, in short, come from the patient himself. But what if it just isn't there? I mean with you, the person suffering from fatness. What if there is inadequate motivation? Deep down you are really convinced that you are sick. You even know that the illness is destroying your life. You know that help and change are possible—but not for you, because you just don't care enough about yourself. You just don't care much about yourself one way or the other. I mean, what the hell, you're not that important. What difference does it make what happens to you? You're a lost cause; you've given up, resigned.

Well, there's one little bit of salesmanship that can sometimes tip the scale in the right direction. Let's say you can't do it for yourself. Well, how about those around you? How do you feel about them? Is there anybody you feel something for? Come now—someone? If there's nobody, get psychiatric help at once! Believe me, there's something radically wrong. But somebody—a daughter or son, a husband or wife, a loved one, somebody! Well, how about doing it for him, for her, for them? They will miss you if you die. Children do need mothers and fathers. How about doing it for them? Sure, it would be better to do it for you. But since you can't, why not at least begin by doing it for them. Do it for them until you see some results. Results—thinness—will encourage you to go on for them and for you as well. Results will improve your self-respect, your self-esteem, a most precious commodity in stimulating motivation and in dynamiting you out of your lethargy and resignation.

So, in the beginning, do it for him, do it for her, do it for them, but make a start, a beginning, and do it! Get going. Eventually you will be doing it for yourself and effectively, too.

Sex, Smoking, and Scruples

Whatever measures can be employed to smooth the way and to make it easier to diet must be seriously considered. We are not interested in a Spartan enterprise of self-deprivation or any kind of unnecessary suffering. We must use every means at our command to arrive at our goal healthfully and comfortably, with a minimum of agonizing.

The fat person is essentially an oral person. Without going deeply into psychiatric theory, and at the risk of oversimplifying, let me explain very simply. The oral person focuses very heavily on his mouth. Much of his activity in life is related to his mouth. He is an eater, a chewer, a talker, in short, a mouth-mover. Now many fat people have isolated themselves from other people. A dislike for how they have come to look has made them intensely shy. You may or may not fit into this category. If you do, you are a person who eats much and talks little. There are varying degrees of the latter mechanism in operation. Some fat people are not aware that they have gradually cut themselves off from other people to a lesser or greater degree, but the fact is that their social lives have been markedly attenuated. Another need of oral people is the need for affection. All people need affection, but oral people need more of it and are greatly affected by its depletion. People need people, and fat people need people most of all, for more than talking purposes, that is. Oral people particularly need to relate to other people; they depend very heavily on other people for a sense of well-being. More often than not fatness has resulted in isolation, anxiety and depression, self-hate, over-eating, and even more isolation. Orally inclined people are also usually sensuous people. They are people whose senses, especially those of touch, taste, and sight, are very keen. They are people who like to imbibe and take in all kinds of sensations via the skin, mouth, eyes, ears. There is nothing good or bad about this. These are simply people who have a large capacity to feel. But often this sensuous quality has been perverted and displaced to the sole area of the mouth and the singular activity of eating.

What am I trying to say? I would like you to enjoy your senses, to reestablish your sensory contact with the world. You will find it most helpful to begin at once to socialize, to talk, to relate, to be active in causes, to visit museums, see plays, see movies. Do things. Be with people.

Sex, especially when it is related to love and loving, will be an asset to your diet. If you are sexually involved, if you have a sexual relationship and a loving relationship at that, then you are lucky indeed. It wouldn't surprise me at all if your sexual activity increases at this time.

Frankly, I believe that this is good. It will provide much of the closeness, love, sensuality, and activity that you need. It will also serve as an outlet for some of the anxiety you will feel in getting rid of a neurotic defense, overeating. If you ask, am I recommending sex? The answer is yes. I am not recommending a big change in your sexual life. I do not, for example, suggest that you suddenly become promiscuous. But if you have been having sex, continue to do so; and if you increase your sexual activity (within reason), this can serve you well during your campaign.

As I explained earlier, this is no time to give up smoking. I do not suggest that you establish this habit if you don't already have it. But if you do smoke, expect a slight increase. Try not to let this increase get out of hand, but don't be hard on yourself if a temporary increase takes place. In my dieting I found that an occasional extra cigar or two helped ease the way.

If your diet and scruples permit, I see no contra-indication to a highball in the evening. This can be something to look forward to. It can be a small social event, and it can make life during this period a little easier and more gracious.

In short, be kind to yourself. Try to increase your engagement in pleasurable activities. Socialize, go to the theater, listen to music, smoke a cigar, love and be loved, go to the beauty parlor, buy a new hat. Do all that you possibly can to raise and to sustain your morale. Do not sit around moping and waiting for things to happen and for weight to be lost. Your diet will take care of the weight; you must take care of yourself. Taking care of yourself will help you take care of your diet. Things will not happen unless you make them happen. So pick up the phone, make contacts, talk to people—especially "real friends"—and help yourself in every way possible to make this period in your life a more pleasant one. This is not the time to save money. I don't suggest you squander it. But this is a good time to indulge yourself. See the play you've been wanting to see. Keep the troops happy but not with food! You needn't watch the scale. This can be most depressing. Get out of the house! Enjoy yourself! Your weight will come down without your concentrating on it. Do take responsibility for your diet, for yourself, and for your enjoyment and well-being. But don't confuse responsibility with concentration. Don't only diet. Enjoy yourself and other people, and trust your diet to do the rest.

By the Group

Group therapy as an adjunct to one's own personal, self-responsible regimen is sometimes very useful. Fat people are usually quite dependent on other people and are very responsive to the reactions of those around them. A group experience can be a good motivating as well as a good supportive force. A group run by a therapist who understands both group dynamics and fatness and its dynamics can be particularly useful. The team cooperative effort and the mutuality of problems and their solutions can be very valuable, especially during difficult times. There are many groups, such as the weight watchers' groups throughout the country, which provide a beneficial atmosphere in which common problems relating to dieting are discussed. In general it is important that these groups, which are not headed by professionals, not attempt deep-insight treatment of any kind. This is not an area for amateurs. It is even more important to guard against the chicanery of bogus professionals who are in fact professional charlatans. Groups headed by qualified people are best; and referral is best sought from your own doctor, county medical society, city health department, or responsible social service agencies such as Catholic Charities and The Jewish Family Service.

The Temptation of Menus

If you are in business or work in an office every day or entertain clients regularly and, in short, must eat out, then you must indeed be careful. However, you can help yourself somewhat. Choose a restaurant that can sensibly cater to your diet without presenting huge temptations. Best of all, make friends with a waiter. Tell him that you are on a diet. Avoid the regular menu and have him suggest foods that are feasible for you. This can be done. I know because I've done it. Don't be shy. This approach will be more than worthwhile.

But what about eating out socially? Don't eat out if you can help it. By all means socialize in every other conceivable way. But eat out as little as possible. What about unavoidable eating out?

First, friends' houses—if you know that you are going to the home of a friendly enemy (more about friendly enemies later), then absolutely make it avoidable. Simply decline dinner invitations. Tell your friendly enemies point blank that you are on a strict diet which you are forbidden (by your physician) to break and that you will arrive after dinner. Do not accept an invitation for dessert! Do eat well (within your diet) before leaving your house in order to avoid the temptation of the midnight snack that will almost certainly be offered. Of course, dinner at real friends' houses will be a different matter. Telling them you are on a diet will help them prepare a meal that is good for you. Real friends will not sabotage your effort.

What about restaurants? Avoid them. It is easier to resist the food that tempting restaurants offer if you don't go to them. Once inside with a menu in hand, you have to be strong indeed to come through unscalded. Try to save eating in restaurants for vacation periods; even then remember that these are times to maintain weight, not to gain it. If, however, going to a restaurant is unavoidable, then once again your friendly waiter can be all important. The people with whom you go will be most important, too. Friendly enemies and a rich gourmet menu are an almost impossible combination to fight successfully. Fish houses will of course be easier to cope with than gourmet French restaurants. But again, if you can, eat at home only or, at least, eat as much as possible at home. Eat well—that is, sociably, graciously, and enjoyably, but do it on safe home grounds. You can enjoy eating out after you have arrived at your goal. Even then care must be exercised. Beware the desserts!

Vitaminizing

What I want to say about vitamins is short but so important that I am using a separate chapter.

Consult your doctor!

There are very few people suffering from vitamin deficiency. However, such deficiency can exist even though you have been eating yourself into fatness for years. On the other hand, your reducing diet may easily be providing you with an adequate vitamin intake. In any case you won't know unless you ask your doctor. This is a most important factor. Vitamin deprivation is serious. Overvitaminizing is just as serious, and self-medicating is just plain foolish. If the doctor who treats himself is treating a fool, a nondoctor who treats himself is treating an even bigger fool. So—you're no fool—ask your doctor. That's what he's there for. Do not take an all-purpose vitamin or miracle vitamins (vitamin A, B, C, D, or E)—ask your doctor. He may feel that you need a multivitamin, a single vitamin, or no vitamin at all. Do listen to him or get yourself a new doctor and listen to him!

The Dietetic Palate

We must not confuse the use of drugs with the use of dietetic foods and aids. Drugs kill the vital sense of responsibility for self that we so desperately need to lose weight and, more important, to maintain that loss later. Drugs serve as a force outside of ourselves and as such shift the center of gravity from us, where it belongs, to the outside. Dietetic foods have no such effect. On the contrary, they help us to exert ourselves in the quest for self-help and self-responsibility. They ease the way, which we certainly appreciate, for we are, as much as possible, against pain.

The variety of sugar-free, low-calorie foods is vast. The department stores and health-food stores are loaded with delicious things, and there is no reason why you can't have them. Such foods will help a great deal in the preparation of ammunition food as well as in the preparation of your diet. Saccharin, artificial sweeteners, and dietetic whipped creams, candy, and cookies will help a great deal should you crave sugar. The choice of dietetic foods is great. There are ersatz whipped creams, candies, desserts, chocolates, puddings, and fruits, and the list goes on and on. There are also any number of recipes that can be easily followed by your wife (a good friend, I hope?), and many people have, on their own, come up with some wonderfully creative dishes that really tempt the palate.

I have had dietetic frappes, malteds, and fruit drinks, with the help of these low-calorie products and just a few ice cubes and a blender, that almost passed for the real thing; the results were no more than 40 calories each. So do make use of what is available, and ease the way as much as possible.

Take Tea for Comfort

No, I do not have any financial interest in the tea industry and I am not Chinese or English. But the Chinese have a good thing in tea. Like them, I consider tea something special. It is not ammunition food and it is not emergency food. I think of it as comforting food. First it's calorie-free and it can keep the mouth going and swallowing. (Keeping the mouth going is all important for fat people.) Also, tea can be drunk warm or cold, having a comforting effect in winter or a refreshing effect in summer. Since tea contains caffeine, it definitely gives a little lift. Tea tastes good taken with any one of a number of artificial sweeteners, and when you get used to it, it tastes even better straight. Most of all, though, drinking tea provides something to do.

Tea is easy to prepare, and for me both preparing it and drinking it have a comforting effect. Perhaps this is due to my own early associations of always seeing the ready teapot my mother kept going for friends who might arrive from the cold. In any case I find it comforting to drink tea, especially during periods of fatigue and the pressure and vicissitudes of dieting.

It is important to have a comforting food on hand that can be quickly prepared—fat people are most receptive to comfort, of course. If you don't like tea, you can have your own "nontea" tea. It doesn't really matter if it's clear broth, bouillon, sugarless coffee or a coffee substitute—as long as it's calorie-free and it warms your innards.

Cold seltzer with a squeeze of lemon or a sugar-free soda is OK, too, as long as it's a food that warms or cools you in that certain way, that is, as long as it eases you and makes you feel a little cozier about yourself and a little more comfortable. Of course, the "tea" has to be easily available. So make up some of your own individual tea, have it on hand, and enjoy it as often and as much as you like with your doctor's approval of course (if it contains caffeine).

The Diet I Like Best

I promised you that this is not a diet book and it isn't. I'm not going to tell you which diet to pursue. Your doctor is best suited to tell you that. But I want to tell you the kind of dieting I like best because it has worked so well for me and because I feel that it is physiologically sound and safe and psychologically tolerable and tenable.

First, I want to stress this again—see your doctor. Before dieting, it is important to equate your diet with any physical malconditions that may exist. This is especially true for people who suffer from gastrointestinal disorders, including gallbladder conditions, ulcers, colitis, and so forth, as well as for those suffering from such things as diabetes and heart disease.

What follows is an oversimplification because I do not want to get technical. But I think that it will suffice to acquaint you with some pretty good diet principles.

Before we begin, let me say that I feel it is very important that you understand the diet you will be following. By understanding, I do not mean the simple *do's* and *don'ts:* Eat this and don't eat that. I mean that you should get your doctor to explain what the diet is all about, what it consists of, and how and why it works. He may hate me for this, but I really do not expect him to make you a nutritionist. I want you to understand, even in simple terms, because I feel it is vital to your sense of responsibility that you understand what you are doing. Just doing is not enough. I want you to be much more than a mechanical man and, if necessary, to be able to make independent decisions. In short, I want you to be a complete participant in your dieting rather than a compliant puppet. This kind of involvement is important if you are to succeed in this essential work. Now on to the diet principles that I like.

First, it is imperative that you evaluate how active or sedentary you are. This will count much in deciding on the amounts of food you can eat. There is simply no magic formula. A sedentary man (for example, a psychiatrist) needs less food than an active man. He burns up less. An older person needs less food. Chances are that he is less active than he used to be. Contrary to popular opinion, ideally one should become lighter as he becomes older. This will help to stave off some of the infirmities of older age and will prevent complications should any physical difficulty arise. To weigh less is to strain the vital organs less. This particularly pertains to the heart and circulatory system.

An excellent internist recently told me that physiologically one should be lighter as one gets older as a natural progression, all other things being equal. This he explained is due to the fact that the bones lose some of their density with age. In any case the determination of calorie intake will depend to a large extent on sex, size in height and body type, the kind of activity one engages in, and age. Your own doctor can best help you to determine caloric necessity and I said "necessity"!

The diet I like best is the high-protein and low-carbohydrate diet. Fish is an excellent protein food, and the more fish on the diet the better. Of course lean meats and chicken are also high protein. Bread, potatoes, sugar, and spaghetti are just about pure carbohydrate and are taboo. I do not suggest a depletion of carbohydrates forever. The body does require some carbohydrate for good function. But a diet designed for weight loss must include a prohibition on carbohydrates; and the man who was once fat will always have to limit his carbohydrate intake.

Now, what is so wonderful about protein and so villainous about carbohydrate? Protein is not just low in calories. It has a characteristic long known to physiologists and biochemists as the "specific dynamic action of protein." Simply speaking, this refers to the fact that protein acts as a kind of metabolic catalyst. It not only burns itself up very readily but it also stimulates the rapid metabolizing of other foods.

Carbohydrates on the other hand are believed to have the reverse effect. Some latter-day researchers even believe that carbohydrates may be an important factor in the retention of cholesterol in the blood stream, which may eventually lead to arterial degeneration and heart and circulatory diseases. This would indeed make a considerable villain of carbohydrates. So what I recommend is a high-protein, low-carbohydrate diet plus the emergency foods and accessory foods mentioned elsewhere.

There are excellent menus prepared for this kind of diet. I would like to mention the ones devised and given by the New York City Board of Health. People I know have received them upon request and I'm sure that you can, too, or your doctor can certainly get them for you. Please remember that fish is a superb food in any diet, and there are some excellent fish dishes well described in any number of cookbooks.

Magic, Miracles, and Myths

There are loads of magic and miracle diets floating around. A new one periodically makes the rounds, and once again every fat man has a new, easy shortcut cure to try out. Claims of miraculous results and magical techniques, whether properly or improperly linked with the name of a famous doctor or hospital, should be considered with suspicion. A very real danger is possible. Many books written for the public, however, do contain sound advice concerning dietary principles; but beware of "miracles"—they can't be purchased!

Initially, some of these diets may really work. Some of them may even go on working. And some of them may go on working and seriously damaging vital organs. Continued and complete depletion of any of the basic food elements can be damaging to the kidneys, heart, and liver to mention just a few important human structures.

The best diet is one in which vital organs get their vital food requirements, and the depletion that does occur is a depletion of calories. Usually, fat people eat too much food, especially too much high-calorie food. Carbohydrates are a particularly high-calorie food. But even during dieting, carbohydrates must not be completely eliminated or radically curtailed for too long for this can be quite damaging.

A high-protein, low-carbohydrate, low-calorie diet for a short time followed by an increase to normal proportions is usually very effective, but again it is only OK if your doctor says so! Otherwise, this diet can have the same effect for you as a gimmicky magic diet. And, gimmicky diets either don't work, or they do work for a while and then don't work, or they have very short lasting results; above all they can be dangerous. So stay away from magic. Let your doctor advise you and put you on a sensible low-calorie diet best suited for your particular health needs.

Help! I'm Starved!

Emergency: I am about to go on a binge.

Quick! Drink two glasses of seltzer, tea, low-calorie soda, coffee substitute, bouillon, or just plain water. Seltzer or a low-calorie soda is best. It blows you up inside and that's what you need. Now eat two pickles (large ones) and a whole cantaloupe (a medium one); then do something very hard. Get out of the house and walk. Here you are, starving, fatigued, filled only by carbonated gas, water, and the equivalent of grass and I ask you to go for a walk. But do it! Get out and walk, walk, walk away from the house—the place where you got fat in the first place; get away from the refrigerator.

Keep going! If things get tough on the way, stop at a luncheonette and without looking at the counter, at the menu, or at dangerous possibilities, quickly order yourself a large, large glass of tomato juice and drink it slowly. If things are still too tough, have a bowl of fresh fruit salad or more cantaloupe and a cup of tea and get out and keep walking. If you have come this far, believe me, victory is within your grasp. Now walk slowly and think about yourself. Look down at your belly. Are you aware of the change? Do you realize that walking is easier than it used to be? Picture yourself and how you look now. Are you passing a store window? Look at it and at your reflection. Look at the nice normal clothes for "normal" people. You are on your way, and who is responsible? You are, that's who. Don't take this lightly. In this emergency situation you need yourself and need to know that you yourself are somebody to reckon with and to take seriously.

By this time that overwhelming urge to eat poison foods is disappearing. You have just about come through an acute emergency. Not only that —you did it in full view of the enemy. That luncheonette contained malteds, chocolates, and sandwiches, and you put them all aside. But the emergency is not quite over. You must go home now, and let me caution you. Going back to the fattening place is the most dangerous time of all. You don't have it beat quite yet. So be careful!

When you get back to the house, either get busy or go to sleep. You are a man who has just been through a great deal. Don't subject yourself to more unnecessary pressures or risk. Remove yourself from the well-wishers who are sitting around eating. Don't sit around alone staring at the four walls or watching television. Read or build a model ship or clean a fish tank or go to sleep. In the morning when you wake up, be fully aware that you have scored a major victory. You have proved that it can be done. Resistance can pay off. You do have self-control and you can do it again if necessary. Not only that—from here on in it's going to get easier.

The Diet Doldrums

There may be times in your regimen when things do not seem to be going well. You will be doing all the prescribed and required things without visible change in the fat "tumor." This is very likely to occur after a sharp initial weight loss and again when you are about two-thirds of your way to your desired goal. Be prepared for these doldrum plateaus so that you don't get unduly discouraged. Usually what is happening is a reshifting of weight distribution and, particularly, a rebalancing of your body's tissue water. The point is that things are in fact happening even though at the moment they may not be demonstrated by your scale or mirror. Stick to the regimen, and you will certainly pass from this doldrum state to a satisfactory period of measurable weight loss.

What generally happens to the body's tissue water is this (again this is an oversimplified explanation): Salt binds liquid, which means that it keeps water in the tissues. A depletion of food and the salt in the food results in a freeing of water so that the kidneys excrete more water through urination. Thus, initial dieting will result in a loss of weight due to water loss. However, as the diet proceeds the salt will gradually be replaced as will the water unless, of course, one remains on a salt-free diet. This is not advisable unless specifically prescribed by a doctor. Many of the so-called reducing pills are nothing more than a combination of diuretics, amphetamines, and hormone substitutes or derivatives. Diuretics are drugs that stimulate the kidneys into greater activity and elimination of water. Thyroxin increases the rate of metabolism—the burning up of food and fat stores. Amphetamines act as mood elevators and appetizer inhibitors. These pills act temporarily, and their usage is usually followed by a rebound water accumulation and depression, resulting in increased eating and weight gain. Such drugs can be dangerous; of course, they should be taken only under the supervision of an ethical, and I repeat ethical, expert in this area.

In any case, there will be doldrums. Be prepared for them and sit them out. Reduced calorie intake must and will work, and the results can be lasting. Do not become discouraged, and do not resort to self-medicating or miracle methods. The body needs time to acclimate—give it that time. Remember, the longer it takes to lose weight, the easier it will be to maintain that loss. But please don't misconstrue this to mean that you should put off dieting.

One final word on this score. If a doldrum period becomes interminable despite faithful, formerly effective dieting, see your doctor. It is possible that your diet needs some modification or that you are accumulating water for a physiological reason. Your doctor may then prescribe appropriate medication. But again remember—pills taken indiscriminately on your own can be a very dangerous affair. The hormonal balance of the body is a very important and delicate one and should be treated with utmost respect.

How to Eat—Graciously

If you are in a culture—and the chances are that you are—where people eat three meals a day, then eat three meals a day. Eat them whether you are hungry or not. Remember the importance of routine; and the routine which best coincides with that of people around you will be the easiest to establish and to maintain. Skipping a meal here and there and then making up for it, or other erratic eating, will not lose weight for you.

A physiologically sound dieting routine as part of a constructive regimen is the only way to lose weight and to sustain the loss. If you are following the New York City Board of Health diet, you will notice that a decent-sized breakfast is prescribed. There are several good reasons for this. People who tend to be depressed find the mornings most difficult. This is also true of fat people who have been defending themselves against depression and anxiety by eating. It's tough to come out of sleep and the dream world and face the ardors of the real world.

Mornings are particularly tough because a whole day of hard work faces us before sleep brings quietness, peace, and dreams again. Facing the day is very difficult when one's metabolism is slowed down from a night's sleeping and fasting. Getting the motor going requires energy, which means food. In addition to the morale-building value of food in the morning, many nutritionists feel that food early in the day serves still another purpose. It acts as a catalyst inasmuch as it starts the metabolizing process going and in the process quickly burns itself up. This quick burning up is further enhanced by the increased energy output of the morning and day hours that follow. Hopefully you exert much more energy in the daytime than you do at night. The price you pay for a good breakfast is relatively small when you consider that your morale is a crucial factor in the attainment of dieting success. The price: eating dinner early (relative to the time you go to bed) and no late eating. Food filling a stomach that has just gone to bed and is half asleep will sit there and turn sluggishly to fat. So eat three meals if prescribed by your doctor and the pattern of your family eating habits. Several small meals are better than fewer large meals. They keep the metabolizing motor going.

But! All early food intake must add up to no more calories than your daily diet calls for. But! All food intake must conform to the diet principle you are following (mine: high protein and low carbohydrates). But! Consume most of your food early; that is, eat so that your food will be digested during waking hours rather than during sleeping hours (good breakfasts and early dinners and no midnight suppers). Now on to another But!

There is a way to eat and a way to eat. If possible, try to eat in pleasant surroundings and among congenial company, and if some ceremonial stuff like nice silverware and nice crystalware is present, so much the better. Good conversation is particularly valuable; for heaven's sake and for your own, eat slowly, chew well, enjoy whatever you are eating, and make the most of it. This is not just whimsy or kidding around, believe me. The fat man is used to wolfing down food just like a wolf—but unlike a wolf, when he is finished he has no memory of having eaten and soon feels empty and ravenous again. For fat people eating has become a piggish thing devoid of charm and concerned only with the momentary filling of the digestive tract. It is our job to restore eating to a convivial social basis. In addition to the obvious increase in social enjoyment, we will also thus satisfy an emotional hunger for sociability, thereby reducing an important tension that has for years been inappropriately handled with food and more food. Also, we will in fact have taken the time to eat slowly and graciously, with people, at a nice table, with nice tableware.

This experience and the ensuing memory of it will give more satisfaction than you think possible in sustaining yourself to the next meal. But! It is most important that the dieter, more than any other person, not eat on the fly, off the top of a desk or standing against a counter. But! The dieter, in eating his required diet food, should whenever possible eat it graciously, socially, slowly, charmingly, festively, and even ceremoniously. For example, if you are about to eat a lettuce, tomato, and sliced egg sandwich (providing your diet permits the two slices of bread), don't! Instead, eat it all as a nicely prepared egg salad with your bread. In other words —you may not be eating much but do eat whatever you eat well.

Trying to deemphasize food by gulping it down quickly without looking at it won't work. Eat what you are supposed to eat and make the most of it. This kind of eating is really eating like a lord, since you will be working in the interest of yourself and hopefully will be lord of yourself. So —enjoy it and even relish it!

On Walking Away from the Table

Yes, it's true that it is a shame to waste food. It is also true that people are starving in India. It would be nice if you could send the excess food on your table to India. But you can't. However, this does not mean that you have to eat it. There is an alternative. Let other people eat it or just throw it away. Stop functioning as a human garbage can. Food in excess of your diet is waste. Throw it in the waste can if other people don't want it. The human garbage can phenomenon is particularly prevalent among mothers but it also exists in fathers and just plain other people. Are you one of these people?

If you've paid money to see a movie that turns out to be a lemon, do you sit through it anyway or do you walk out? I hope you walk out. It's bad enough to have misspent the money, but it's even worse to torture yourself for it. Of course, the same applies to food. The fact that you have spent money and bought too much food does not mean you have to poison yourself with it.

Now when you have had enough—within the

limits of your diet—get up and leave the table. You've heard this before and perhaps it sounded silly. But there's nothing silly about it. For a food addict to sit and stare at a table loaded with goodies creates unnecessary temptation and a situation fraught not only with danger but also with destructive and useless torture. Therefore, get up and leave the table and, if necessary, the room. This may not fit in with the social amenities but it will fit in with your most urgent needs and self-interest. Forget about the food that is still there. Let others take care of it or throw it away! Forget about the waste and the hundred other rationalizations. Next time, buy less, but this time (and every time there is excess food), use the garbage can—not you! You are not a walking food disposal unit. You are a human being on the way to being healthier and more attractive.

Your Evening Evaluation

This is just a short chapter to tell you to spend a few minutes each evening before you go to sleep evaluating the day, dietwise and otherwise. Now I don't mean for you to get started on an obsessive evening binge that will both demoralize you and keep you from sleeping. I certainly do not recommend a presleep self-beating that will contribute to nightmares. I simply feel that it may be of value to make a simple evaluation of how the day has gone with an eye toward possible prophylaxis and improvement the next day. Were there any difficult periods? How did you get through them? Are there any areas in which there can be improvement tomorrow? Areas that should best be avoided as too tempting? Were there any significant victories? How was your morale? Is there any way to improve it tomorrow? Did you have too much spare time? Weekends are particularly tough; have you any ideas on additional interesting activities? Are things getting easier? How about more social involvement in other than eating activities? Is there an eating place near the office best avoided to-morrow?

An evening and weekend evaluation can be of value, but please remember to use it constructively and not in the service of self-punishment. Keep in mind that self-hate will always remain your No. 1 enemy!

Apples, Aspirin, Amour

There are side reactions and complications associated with dieting. It is best to be aware of them and, as much as possible, to be prepared for them. This will help dispel fear, discouragement, and failure. The following is a small list of a few complications I have encountered. Expect more of them. Each of us has his or her special brand of symptomatology that makes itself felt when we are depleted of the dope we've been taking for years.

Constipation: This can be distressing, painful, and a blow to the morale. Less input will result in less output. Most diets will result in a sharp decrease in food intake and a consequent decrease in fluid in food; these, as well as fat depletion, make constipation a very common problem. Unless contra-indicated by your diet or doctor, you can do the following: Drink plenty of water—at least six glasses a day—especially in the summer when one perspires a great deal. Eat plenty of green vegetables—lettuce, kale, beet ends, spinach, and so forth. They are all low in calories, too. Eat two whole *raw* apples a day, just two raw apples, neither baked nor scraped.

If any day passes in which you have not had a movement, take a spoonful of mineral oil that night. If another day passes, take another spoonful of mineral oil plus one spoonful of milk of magnesia. If your constipation is chronic, ask your doctor if it is advisable for you to take a tablespoon of mineral oil every night for the duration of your diet. If constipation becomes severe enough to cause an impaction, use an enema consisting of a small amount of warm water. Or, perhaps, your doctor will recommend a disposable enema preparation now available at all drugstores. Then have some on hand at all times. They can save you a great deal of pain and distress.

Headache, fatigue, mild depression, transient weakness, listlessness, insomnia: All of these can be initial symptoms in dieting and all can be both psychological and physiological in origin. We are removing an old well-engraved defense, and as a result anxiety and its concomitant symptoms (the above) will in large or small part surely occur. In taking in less food, we are also depleting the blood stream of much of the glucose we have become used to. The initial response to this "lack" of sugar can produce a vast myriad of symptoms singly or in combination. However, these symptoms will pass and you will become acclimated. You are not dying; therefore, don't, whatever you do, look to food for succor. If you are weak and tired, lie down, take a nap, relax in a warm bath; then go out and enjoy yourself. These symptoms will pass. Give yourself a chance, and meanwhile make use of your prepared supply of ammunition and comforting foods.

Of course, if you have any propensity for neurotic symptoms, and who hasn't, initial dieting may bring it out. I am not talking about severe anxiety and depression. That would obviously require psychiatric help. But if some of your neurotic habits become accentuated, don't be hard on yourself. Ride them out. They will pass along with your "tumor."

Increased or decreased libido: This can go either way. The depletion of food and sugar can result initially in great fatigue and concurrent loss of sexual desire. This is not evidence of early impotence or frigidity. It is a transient symptom and will pass. Sometimes, however, a deprivation of food will lead to the displacement of interest from eating to sex. Also, many people make use of sex in handling their anxieties. The closeness that sex brings, the relaxation, and even the fatigue, all have ameliorative effects. If there is an increase in sexual appetite during this period, enjoy it by all means.

There is no point in adding to the list. Sex is a pleasant point of departure. Suffice it to say that you are liable to have all kinds of symptoms —headaches, restlessness, and so forth. You will also get attacks of food craving. Take an aspirin if you have to but stick to your diet! This period of initial difficulty will pass. Be prepared for it! Don't be alarmed! Things will get better!

The Night Eaters

As with all illnesses, manifestations and degrees of illness will vary in different patients. The most serious form of fatness is often manifested in compulsive night eating. The victim of this form of overeating feels compelled to awaken one or more times during the night to load up on a vast quantity of food. This occurs nearly every night, regardless of how much food was eaten during the day. This manifestation is almost always evidence of a serious eating compulsion based upon severe anxiety and a poor anxiety tolerance.

Unless treated, night eaters often eat their way into a very early grave, for they have been known to be overweight by as much as 200 pounds. Many of these people suffer from chronic heart failure as well as from lung embarrassment, which leaves them gasping for air in the reclining position. Ideally this condition should be treated both physically and psychiatrically. Many of these poor people require hospitalization as a lifesaving device. This form of the illness does not occur suddenly. It becomes chronic and malignant over an extended period of time. The longer it persists, the poorer will be the prognosis.

If you demonstrate evidence of night eating, do something about it immediately! If you get up for an occasional stuffing session at night and if these sessions are becoming more frequent, then you are in great danger. It would be of great benefit to you to seek both physiological and psychiatric assistance.

Initially you ought to see a competent internist who can evaluate your total condition, especially that of your heart, lungs, and blood pressure. He may well refer you to a competent psychiatrist, and together both of them can evaluate with you the merits of a possible short period of hospitalization. Hospitalization can be of benefit in the evaluation of your total physical condition. It can also serve to remove you from destructive forces in your environment. Primarily, though, it can start you on a disciplined diet under the supervision of trained personnel.

Of course, this discipline will come from outside of you and as such will not be as effective in promoting your sense of responsibility as if it came from you alone. But it is a beginning, a very important beginning, which can save you from a severely malignant condition and can possibly save your life. Hospitalization can often start the therapeutic process off sufficiently so that the patient can carry on later without the hospital. In these cases the added support of psychotherapy, especially with a psychiatrist trained in psychoanalysis, can be invaluable. In these cases psychotherapy may offer the only prophylaxis in preventing recurrent attacks and the necessity of further hospitalization.

If you are a neophyte night eater, do not wait until you have gained another hundred pounds. It can happen, but don't let it. Do something about it now! What I have suggested is a radical treatment but night eating is a most serious condition. Don't wait until it has become a full-blown chronic affair. Seek professional consultation now!

Beware of Friendly Enemies

Beware of your well-meaning friends and relatives. Many, many of them (not all, of course) will be serious deterrents to your goal. Enemy action will range from the most subtle to the most blatant sabotage. Let me explain.

Nearly all people have a peculiar but very important characteristic in common: They are afraid of the unfamiliar. They will go to fantastic lengths to avoid the unknown. In so doing, people will exert great effort to maintain the status quo. This even applies to people in pain. I know that it sounds peculiar, but people who have been sick for years and who do in fact wish to be well will at the same time be terribly frightened of changing to a healthier state.

The psychiatrist will tell you how his patients cling tenaciously to their neuroses. They want to get well, but at the same time they have a great need to retain the status quo and to keep away from unfamiliar ground, however healthy. The resistance and obstacles placed in the way of change and progress can be enormous. Scientists and social scientists have encountered this resistance only too often. A large part of the lives of such people as Pasteur, Freud, Ben-Gurion, Semmelweis, was spent overcoming resistance to change. Now this resistance is particularly true in people's relationships with each other. Very often this process goes on unconsciously; sometimes it is fairly close to the surface and can be perceived quite readily.

In any case, people will fight the possibility of any change in their fellows or associates which may make for a change in role. They want constellations to remain fixed and each member to move in his expected orbit, fixed and predictable. You have all heard people say, "So-and-so is getting so well educated, soon he won't bother with us," "He's becoming such a big shot," or "She looks so good she soon won't need us." While people do sincerely want the best for their fellows, they are threatened by change and will resist it and even sabotage it.

Now what has your role been? Of course there have been many facets to your life and influences in your social and familial circle. But one of your principal roles has been that of the fat man. Many of the people around you will make every effort to keep you in that role. If you confront them with this statement, they will be insulted, deny it vigorously, or call you crazy. But they will go right on sabotaging your effort. What does this mean in practical terms? It means that you must be prepared for the onslaught and must at all costs withstand it. The more you believe in your cause and in yourself, the easier your resistance will be. But be prepared. Here are some examples of enemy action.

1. Whenever you open the refrigerator or

come to the table, there will be foods there that have always tempted you. This will be especially true when you are at a low point and are most vulnerable. Your wife, mother, sister, and friend are unconscious experts at picking up your more vulnerable moods. They will often recognize one long before you do.

2. There will be people who insist that you eat out. They will tell you that you can eat diet food and then guide you to restaurants offering the most tempting and fattening foods—all "poison" for you.

3. There will be the force feeders who will pressure you endlessly to eat something—"a little something at least." "So go off your diet just this once, just for a little while." "Give yourself a little break." "Don't be so hard on yourself." "After all, a little moderation is a good thing."

4. Beware of statements like these: "You are thin enough already." "You look so pale, so pinched." "You won't lose more off your belly anyway." "I think you are overdoing it." "For God's sake, you'll get tuberculosis." "Good God, don't be so compulsive about this thing." "Know something? I liked you better the other way. You looked more jolly." "You seem so moody. I think you've dieted enough already." "You are so damned irritable—eat and be happy."

5. Everything is going well when your wife will slip just a little bit of potatoes or a sliver of apple pie or chocolate cake on your plate. After all, she feels sorry for you and she can see that you crave a little something, especially since everybody else is eating like crazy and the pie is so good and it's just a little piece anyway, so how can it matter?

The list can go on and on. There is no point in further enumeration. Each of you will undoubtedly be in contact with your own particular kind of sabotage specialist. I do want to say this, however: In a temper tantrum, many fat people will go on an acute eating binge to get even with someone and everyone. This is a very special kind of attack, unfortunately very common and sometimes very subtle. It goes like this: "I'll show you. I'll really louse myself up. I'll get so fat you won't be able to stand me and then you'll be sorry." Of course, when you cut your nose off, the hole is in your own face. Another side of the same coin is unconscious compliancy on the part of the fat person. The compliant person will do nearly anything to please another person. In this case the fat man would rather eat than displease a feeder. Remember, your first duty is to yourself. You cannot please everyone. Change the status quo and please yourself. Nobody is closer to you than you. You have to be with you all of the time, and it would be nice if your constant companion was thin, healthy, and attractive.

So please be a friend to yourself. You need you. If the people around you sense that you are absolutely dedicated to your cause, they may well come over to your side. If nothing else, your strong and good resolve will help to block and mitigate their unconscious and not so unconscious sabotage. Who knows? Perhaps some of them will even become real friends, and some may even go on a much needed diet themselves.

Allies to the Cause

Real friends are people who will get your message without your really trying. It is not hard for them to know where you are going or how you are going to get there. Not only won't they create roadblocks but they will help you however they can along the way. These people believe in you, in the possibility of change, in your changing, and in your ability to reach your goal. These friends have a keen appreciation for the difficulty of your job, the worthiness of it, and the wonderful effort you are making. They will not pressure you to do more or prod you or censure you or pity you or patronize you. Though they will be there and will support your cause, they will also respect you as an adult and as such will appreciate that this is your job and that the effort must come essentially from you.

Your real friend-wife will prepare the proper foods, not tempt you with poison foods; she will readily sacrifice eating out in "dangerous spots;" she will make an effort to understand your diet; and she will even tolerate your moodiness and irritability if necessary.

Do suggest to your immediate family that they read this book. Their understanding of the scope and nature of the work that you, a loved one, are engaged in can be a valuable asset.

On occasion there will be more than one person in the family who is attempting to lose weight. You may even inspire someone who never thought of it to do likewise. This, of course, is a valuable opportunity for you to become a real friend. Eating with someone who is also dieting is not only more congenial but also much easier. A mutually constructive effort can be most helpful and supportive to all parties concerned. In this mutual-help society, you will undoubtedly also find that you are your own best friend. Make use of this friendship. Learn to know yourself, to appreciate yourself, to get closer to yourself, and to have a higher esteem for yourself and your accomplishments.

Your Body Image

In an earlier chapter I spoke of how we see ourselves. Now this is all important, so let me elaborate. Each of us unconsciously and very often quite consciously has an image of how he looks. The image varies from the way he really looks to great deviations from the actuality. I remember a woman patient who worked as a model and was very beautiful indeed. Her image of herself was that of an ugly duckling, and no amount of reassurance could sway her from this self-concept. This body image is formed very early in life and evolves slowly and carefully, remaining extremely resistant to change. The body image is extremely important because it contributes a great deal to the feeling of self and to one's general identity. The body image, or how we see ourselves, is most intimately connected with our sense of physical identification.

More often than not we are convinced and remain convinced that people see us the way we see ourselves even though the picture they see may be completely different from the one we have in mind. To further complicate things, we often project our own body-image concepts and reactions in viewing other people. This in large part accounts for the completely diverse descriptions several people might give when describing the same person.

I have met fat people who are truly not aware that they are fat because they still retain an early engraved thin image of themselves. I have also met thin people who have been thin for years and who are still on rigid diets because they see themselves as fat. These distortions due to body image often account for some women buying clothes that are much too small for them while others buy clothes that are much too large.

Obviously, the body image will play an enormous role in your life as a fat person becoming thin. It is imperative that you question yourself and determine what your concept of your physical self is and how closely it compares with reality. This is the only way in which you can determine how great your problem is in terms beyond the scale. I speak here of terms that you will understand emotionally—deep in your guts where it counts.

I spoke earlier about how people cling tenaciously to the familiar. This is especially true of the body image. This need to cling to an old, however sick, concept of ourselves can offer considerable resistance to change and thus to our cause. Familiarity with this problem of body image and the need to cling to it as well as familiarity with reality and with our goal will help to overcome this resistance and enhance our chances for success.

Some understanding of this concept will also

enable us in part to change our body image commensurate with actual body change. We cannot expect a total body-image change inasmuch as this image is extremely well ingrained and is linked to many personality traits we have had since earliest times. For a greater change to take place, psychoanalysis would be necessary and even then a complete change would not be possible. But can anything in life ever be complete other than death? In any case, understanding the concept of body image and your very own body image can put you in ever so much better contact with reality. Nothing serves our purpose better than reality. Knowing who and what we are helps us immeasurably in becoming who and what we want to be.

Success—and Maintenance

You are at your goal! Congratulations! You've done it. Arrived! No longer fat. Thin, once fat, now thin, actually thin. If you don't believe it, look in the mirror, full-length, please. Thin, can you see it? Can you believe it? You think you still look heavy? That you can be a little thinner? Don't believe it! You are playing tricks on yourself. At this point, this is a common illusion. Your old image of the fat man is playing tricks on you. Your new image is not firmly implanted yet. This will take time, at least several months and even more! Now do not succumb to temptation! I mean to continue to diet—to get thinner and thinner and thinner. It won't change the fat feeling. At this point nothing will change it but time. You need time as a thin person to come around to feeling like one and seeing yourself as one. Getting too thin will only make you dried out, ugly, and older; and it can be downright dangerous. Imagine somebody warning you about being too thin—a sure sign that you have arrived.

Well, now that the congratulations are over—back to work.

Please remember that as a formerly fat person (of several years' duration), you are something like the former alcoholic. The fat "tumor" is gone, but this is not true of your susceptibility and addiction to food. I believe that this—shall we call it *sensitivity* to food—will always exist. Be aware of it! Accept it and respect it. This reality is all important in the prevention of future fat "tumors." Now all this is not easy. But getting thin was not easy either and you did it. So let's not take your newly emancipated status as a thin person lightly. As a matter of fact, you now have to guard it and guard it zealously against the encroachment of fat. So you say, "What kind of emancipation is this? All my life I have to watch out." Well, it is an emancipation. As your body image conforms with your new bodily dimensions, you will begin to appreciate that you are emancipated and a thousand times freer in areas much more important than food. I'm talking about relating to other people—economically, sexually, socially. From here on in it's going to be much easier—even fun. Imagine having the so-called (and questionable) ebullient disposition of the fat man and the good looks of the thin man. Can't miss.

But on to food. A fat man is never free. But then who is? Complete freedom doesn't exist. Even a free man living in a land that guarantees freedom of speech is not permitted to yell "fire" in a crowded theater. Well, you can't just eat. I mean that you can't just eat wildly and indiscriminately; the truth is you never will have wild abandon in your eating—not if you want to remain thin. Oh, sure, now and then you may allow yourself tiny periods of complete freedom.

But you must make sure that these periods remain tiny and encapsulated. They must never become chronic and malignant. Even more dangerous now will be the tendency to slip gradually into a larger and larger eating habit and to ignore or rationalize a tiny but steady weight gain. Now your eating, your post-diet diet, must not become a state of eating anarchy. While you will not have complete freedom, you will have greater freedom. This new freedom, however, will really be based on the knowledge that you have been very sick and have the potential for great sickness—fatness. It will therefore consist of a wider latitude but a disciplined and calculated latitude designed to keep you happy and happily thin. This maintenance diet should be at least as carefully considered and constructed as your reducing diet. This is definitely no time for the patient to abandon his doctor. You can now make the best use of his knowledge in constructing a diet that is right for you. Such a diet will of course be based on your individual health needs, your body type, your daily activity, and your caloric needs. The diet that will be easiest to handle will be the one most closely resembling the norm, that is, the one that the people you are around are eating. Beware and doubly beware if you are living with a lot of resigned fatties. Unfortunately, sick fat people sometimes like company and inadvertently will attempt to seduce you back into their fat fraternity. Also, the most successful maintenance diet will probably be based on the principles of your reducing diet. They have worked; therefore they are good; and you are now used to them so this should be relatively easy. Of course, the maintenance diet will have modifications, including greater leeway and occasional divergences from too rigorous a regimen. For example, it may be all right now to have ice cream once a week for dessert. But, if it's to be once a week, keep it at once a week. If you find that you can't, then please get back to your doctor and substitute for the ice cream a treat less addictive to you. Once again I would like to stress the value of having dieted slowly. Because you have taken a considerable time to lose weight, both your psychology (regarding food) and your stomach have been considerably reduced. Therefore, the maintenance diet should feel like more than enough. It may therefore be wise to increase your intake gradually rather than sharply, but do not slip into an escalating, uncontrollable increase. Be especially careful, and this is most important, during periods of stress. Remember that, despite your recent victory, you have subjected yourself to years of conditioning in which stress and depression were handled with food. So be very, very careful at times when things aren't going just right. We must all encounter bumps in the road—don't handle yours with a big fat food regression.

Now during your maintenance period—the rest of your life—the scale will be essential. This will be your most reliable instrument in determining success, danger, and potential maintenance failure. Make sure your scale is a good one. Use it once a day, preferably in the morning before breakfast and before dressing, in any case consistently with regard to food, clothing, and time of day. Use it as a prophylaxis and you will not regret it. Here is one suggestion. Let us say that your correct weight is 175 pounds. Then bring your weight down to 170 pounds. If you continue to weigh between 170 and 175 pounds, a fluctuation radius of five pounds, then your maintenance diet is working. If you drop below 170, an increase is in order. If you rise above 175—and I mean even 175.1—then immediately begin your reducing diet again. But to give you ample leeway, do not go back to your maintenance diet until you go down to 172, i.e., three pounds below your desired goal. At 172 pounds, go back on the maintenance diet, this time slightly reduced. Follow this rule carefully, and you will never get back into serious trouble. Eventually you will become so well stabilized that there will be practically no fluctuation at all. Use the scale daily and the latter simple calculation from here on in. Of course, a very small person can apply the same principle, using a smaller fluctuating radius.

Well, you are on your way. Again I want to congratulate you. I won't wish you luck. It's not luck that brought you this far. It's self and self-esteem and you have proved that you've got plenty of that. Continue to apply it, I mean your self-esteem, and you will be fine. And by the way, welcome to the fraternity of thin people formerly fat.

Glossary

The following new or almost new terms are used throughout this book. This is to provide a common language for descriptive purposes. The terms are simple.

Acute binge: A short period of indiscriminate, voracious eating.

Acute emergency: The verge of going on a food binge.

Ammunition food: Food that can be eaten in any quantity without weight gain. These foods should always be available. They include such foods as mushrooms, celery, carrots, string beans, dill or kosher pickles, brussels sprouts, sauerkraut, and so forth.

Chronic binge: A deteriorated acute binge where control is lost and the person has rededicated himself to the growth of the "tumor."

Comforting food: Food that is special in its comforting capacity and fat people need comfort. These foods include tea, coffee, bouillon, dietetic sodas.

Danger spot: A restaurant offering "poison" foods—usually a great place to eat.

D Day: Day of diet commencement.

Doldrums: A period in which no weight loss is discernible. But sit it out—it's happening.

Emergency food: To be used when a binge is imminent. Unlike ammunition food, not to be eaten indiscriminately but rather to be used effectively and as a means of producing a stopgap. Such foods include a large hamburger, a steak, half a chicken, fish, a piece of hard cheese, a cantaloupe.

Excess "poison" foods: Whipped cream, cake, rich desserts, and so forth.

Fatty: A person suffering from simple fatness, uncomplicated by any thyroid dysfunction. This is a most serious sickness whether the person has admitted it or not.

Fat "tumor": That extra weight in the form of fat wherever it may be. The "tumor" is generally spread all over the body with special predilection for the hips, belly, buttocks, thighs, arms, neck, and chin.

Friendly enemy: A saboteur of our cause.

Goal unit or segment unit: This will be a unit of never more than 20 pounds strived for in order to earn a vacation.

Maintenance: After arrival at ultimate goal and for the rest of your life, during which time you will maintain your new-found state of health.

Maintenance diet: That diet which will sustain your new-found status without gain or loss.

"Poison" foods: Food that you know will spread the "tumor." This can be qualitative or quantitative. There are foods that are loaded with fatty possibilities. Then there is eating on a scale so massive that it will produce fatness regardless of the particular food, unless it is ammunition food.

Real friend: Anyone with faith in you who will not deter you from your work.

Scale: An object for measuring weight. It is more important to use each day after arrival at maintenance than during dieting.

Temptation: Food not on your diet.

Toughest period: Any period that is particularly difficult. These are the periods immediately following the end of an acute emergency and the period immediately following arrival at the ultimate goal.

Ultimate goal: The point at which you arrive at your correct weight.

Vacation: At the end of each goal unit, a period of one month in which the winning diet is abandoned for the maintenance diet.

Victory: Any reestablishment of control during an emergency or a binge.

Winning diet: The diet you and your doctor arrived at for you to lose weight sensibly and slowly; the diet is, of course, commensurate with your state of health. This is one time when if you lose you win.

Working units: From 10 to 20 percent of the total "tumor" at any given time. This will be the unit you will contemplate in the work that has to be done.

Questions and Answers

"Everybody in my family is fat. Could this tendency be inherited?"

While glandular patterns and anomalies and subsequent malfunctions can run through families, these are relatively rare conditions. The chances are that your family has bad eating habits which have been passed on from generation to generation for a good many years. In short, overeating can be learned and can become a family way of life.

"Is fatness psychosomatic?"

This depends on your definition of the term *psychosomatic*. In my frame of reference, I would say yes. Psychological disturbances cause overeating, and here the body or somatic lesion is fatness, thus warranting the term *psychosomatic.*

"Do men and women gain weight in the same places?"

Sometimes, but generally men tend to gain above the belt line while women tend to gain below the belt line as well as in the hips, buttocks, and breasts.

"Does exercise help get rid of stretch marks?"

While there is some justification for the use of exercise in helping to prevent and get rid of stretch marks, in most cases exercise will have no effect. I, along with several of my friends who are dermatologists, feel that stretch marks are related to the amount of natural resiliency one's skin does or does not have. This is an inherited characteristic related to the amount of fibrous tissue in the skin. The only prophylaxis I know is not to stretch the skin by getting terribly fat in the first place and especially not to get fat and thin, fat and thin, again and again but rather to attain and sustain thinness.

"Why must I call myself sick to be effective?"

Because if you are fat you are sick, and you must admit and accept this fact in order to be utterly realistic. Reality is a prime necessity in the treatment of sickness, especially that which relates in any way to a psychological disorder.

"Isn't it the style in some cultures to be fat?"

Yes, and in other cultures it is the style to hallucinate, to castrate, to disfigure, to mutilate, and to tattoo, and these activities are probably all safer than being fat. These cultures, may I say, have little concern about elevated blood pressure, arteriosclerosis, coronary heart disease, and strokes which well may result in your spending the rest of your short life as a paralytic in a wheelchair.

"How can I motivate my fat husband?"

This is exceedingly hard. Your good relationship with him will be all important. You must treat him kindly, firmly, and confidently. This confidence must be in yourself as well as in him. You might try to have a serious sit-down discussion in which you indicate to him his importance to you and the rest of the family and his future state of health. Perhaps if he cannot do it for himself initially, he will start by doing it for you and the children. Nagging will not help. Once he has started, your cooperation will be of utmost importance.

"How about fat little babies that are supposed to be so healthy?"

They're not. Most pediatricians agree that it is an extremely unhealthy practice to stuff and fatten a child and most psychiatrists agree that this early food orientation can be disastrously carried on into later life.

"But I have a friend with whom I eat now and then who gorges himself with beer, no less, and remains thin. He has no thyroid trouble. So?"

He is probably a sporadic eater. When he eats, he eats a good deal but he seldom eats; that is, he eats fewer meals. All in all, you can be sure that he ingests fewer calories than you do and certainly not more than he needs in order to sustain his weight.

"When I don't eat, I get so moody. What can I do?"

Moodiness can connote conditions ranging

from transient blueness to deep depression. If keeping active, renewing old acquaintances, interesting yourself in new enterprises, and such, do not help, you might consider a psychiatric consultation.

"Is there such a thing as a naturally fat person?"

There are naturally large, broad-boned people, but there are no naturally fat people. Fatness takes stuffing, and stuffing is not a natural phenomenon.

"Why is there so much prejudice against fat people?"

Gluttony and its concomitant sins have a longstanding place in human history, including early biblical origins. I think, however, that most people are contemptuous of fatties because obesity indicates a lack of self-control plus a narcissistic preoccupation with self-stuffing. If an overwhelming prejudice exists it is almost always concerned with oneself and often with one's self-image which turns out to be that of a fat man. In short, this prejudice is a self-hate projected to the individual who most reminds the hater of his own feared and loathsome self.

"My husband says that he wants me to get thin, but then he brings home cake and all kinds of goodies for himself and the kids and tells me that I must exert self-control. Is he a friendly enemy?"

He is a friendly enemy and then some.

"What do I do when I invite people to dinner at my home?"

Eat your diet only before their arrival and then go on to feed them.

"I simply can't get to bed early and when I try I feel so hungry I can't fall asleep. What can I do?"

Prepare lots of OK foods (sour pickles, mushrooms, cantaloupe, brussels sprouts, celery stalks, carrot sticks) and use them as needed. Try to go to sleep a little bit earlier each night until you have succeeded in changing your sleep pattern.

"Are all fat people psychiatric cases? And if so, don't they all need psychiatric treatment?"

People are people and not cases. Many fat people suffer from personality problems, and fatness is often only one of many symptoms. Nearly all people can gain from some form of psychotherapy, but some people *need* therapy. Others can improve without therapy. This applies to fat, thin, and medium alike.

"From a psychiatric point of view, what is the chief force behind pure overeating and getting fat?"

There is no chief force. There are many forces and factors and they vary from individual to individual. It would take many months of careful analysis to understand the particular disturbance pattern of a given individual. But the one basic generator of fatness as well as nearly all other psychiatric symptoms is anxiety.

"Why do some people 'eat' when they are anxious and depressed while others 'fast'?"

Again this can only be explained in terms of each individual's psychological makeup and background. This makeup is based on one's unique individual history from infancy on up and is particularly affected by one's early familial relationships and environmental teachings.

"Why are fat people as a rule jollier than thin people?"

I don't know that this is a rule at all. It may even be an outdated cliché. In my professional experience fatness has for the most part made for much misery. If a fat person is jolly it is for factors other than and despite his fatness. However, it is possible that people who are jolly in the first place tend to be big eaters and that some are susceptible to becoming excessive eaters. However, I don't feel that there is enough solid evidence to warrant conclusions correlating fatness and good-naturedness.

"Are the circus fat man and woman freaks or mutations?"

Neither. They are fatties, excessive eaters just like other fatties but on an expanded scale. They are, incidentally, engaged in an occupation which is much more dangerous than that of any of their other circus colleagues.

"Are there particular dishes you found satisfying for lunch during your own dieting?"

Chicken, water-packed tuna, scallops, large nonfatty hamburgers, shrimp, and lots of lettuce and tomatoes.

"What did you weigh?"

I am six feet three inches tall and I scaled down from 245 to 195 pounds.

"How come a psychiatrist got fat?"

Psychiatrists are people. People have problems. This is why psychiatrists get analyzed.

"My brother-in-law is enormous. He comes to our house often and heads right for the refrigerator. He doesn't stop nibbling until he leaves. I am not a friendly enemy. What can I do?"

Tell him that you do not want to contribute to his early death. Therefore, "Stay the hell out of my kitchen." Add that he will be most welcome to your food stores when his life is no longer in jeopardy, unless of course you'd rather he stay out.

"What do you think of doctors who give pills for fatness?"

I don't like charlatans in any form, and I certainly don't like medical mass-production methods. The astute and conscientious practitioner who specializes in weight reduction for the treatment of obesity certainly deserves a respected place among the medical specialties. This is a harrowing and complicated disease and is deserving of specialty training and treatment. But this responsible practitioner will never be a simple pill pusher. He knows his patient well, checks his patient carefully, and treats his patient as his unique needs require.

As I've stated in the text, except in very special cases in which immediate heroic methods are needed in order to save a life, I do not favor pills.

They destroy one's much needed sense of responsibility and do not help the ultimate goal of sustained thinness.

"What do you mean by a crash diet?"

A diet designed to lose several pounds quickly. This does not mean starvation and must always be compatible with your state of health. This can only be achieved without danger by the attendance of a competent physician.

"Are milk farms effective?"

Farms, hotels, hospitals, and institutions that are run conscientiously on an efficient dietary plan that considers each individual's needs carefully can be especially useful in starting a therapeutic regimen. However, sustaining success will still ultimately depend on reorientation of one's eating and living. Eating must become a peripheral activity rather than the central-core phenomenon of one's life. Only a real interest in self and a keen awareness of one's own responsibility in this vital matter can produce sustained results.

"I don't quite understand the process of segmenting the 'tumor,' can you explain?"

Since this is a major contribution to sustaining weight loss, I'll gladly explain:

In working on "tumor" reduction on a day-to-day basis, we must *not* think in terms of the total "tumor"—let us say 70 pounds. This is not practical and it can be very demoralizing. Instead, after an initial morale booster of let us say a 10 percent or 7 pound loss resulting from crash dieting, we then think in terms of small working units of 5 to 10 pounds as we watch the overall "tumor" disappear. Meanwhile, we also think in terms of goal units of no more than 20 pounds each. When a goal unit has been reached, in this case a reduction of the original "tumor" from 70 to 50 pounds, we are ready for a thirty day vacation. This period should be one in which the maintenance-diet plan will be employed so that there will be neither weight loss nor gain. After thirty days, there should be a return to dieting again, in terms of working units and another goal unit with another reward vacation period to follow. This should be done until the final goal has been reached and the permanent maintenance diet adopted as a way of life.

After these early experiences of maintaining weight as well as losing it, it will be much easier to continue successfully maintaining your proper weight on a lifetime basis. You will have had time to experience your ability to lose weight; your ability to sustain that loss; and your ability to quickly return to a weight-losing diet when required. You will have attained a new outlook on food as well as an ever changing image of yourself as a thin rather than a fat person.

"Is the psychotherapy of a fat man different from that of anybody else?"

As a symptom complex some special problems and solutions may be necessary in the psychiatric treatment of a fat person. But here, as in the treatment of all people, profound respect for the unique characteristics of each individual patient must always be exercised. Here, as in the treatment of all people, psychotherapy—especially that based on psychoanalytic theory and technique—will aim at basic and deeper symptom-causing problems rather than on symptoms themselves. Treatment, as with nonfat people, will be involved with one's attitude toward one's self, the world, and other people and one's ways of relating to fellow human beings.

"I've been fat and I mean very fat for as long as I remember. Can I really get well?"

Yes. If you really want to, you can really get well.

Ammunition Foods

Keep plenty of these foods handy. They are satisfying and contain very few calories—you can eat all you want!

- beets (and greens)
- broccoli
- brussels sprouts
- cabbage
- cauliflower
- celery
- chard
- cucumbers
- dandelion greens
- gelatin (unsweetened)
- leeks
- lettuce
- mushrooms
- onions
- parsley
- pickles
- radishes
- raw peppers
- sauerkraut
- spinach
- string beans
- tomato juice
- watercress

Comforting Foods

These foods are of relatively low caloric content and are more "filling" than Ammunition Foods. You can't eat *all* you want—but these are great for fighting off that urge . . .

- apples
- apricots
- artichokes
- asparagus
- cantaloupe
- carrots
- chestnuts
- chicken
- cottage cheese
- egg plant
- grapefruit
- lean beefburgers
- lobster
- mussels
- pears
- pot cheese
- scallops
- shrimp
- strawberries
- tangerines
- tomatoes
- veal

. . . and for Special Comfort, drink

bouillon coffee tea

"Poison" Foods

These foods are tagged with this warning label to remind you to keep away from them; they are high in calories and are destructively dangerous to you!

ale
avocado
baked apple (sugared)
baked beans
beer
bread—in excess
butter—in excess
cake
candies
chocolate
cookies
cream
cream cheese
creamed soups
dates
doughnuts
dressings
dried fruits
duck
fat meats
goose
gravies
griddle cakes
ice cream
jams
jellies
macaroni
malted milk
nuts
peanut butter
pie
pizza
spaghetti
sugar—in excess